BABY SIGNING ESSENTIALS

EASY SIGN LANGUAGE FOR EVERY AGE AND STAGE

NANCY CADJAN

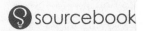 sourcebook

Published by Sourcebooks, Inc.
P.O. Box 4410, Naperville, Illinois 60567-4410
(630) 961-3900
Fax: (630) 961-2168
www.sourcebooks.com

Library of Congress Cataloging-in-Publication Data

Cadjan, Nancy.
  Baby signing essentials : easy sign language for every age and stage / Nancy Cadjan.
    pages cm
  Includes index.
  (trade paper : alk. paper) 1. Nonverbal communication in infants. 2. Sign language acquisition. 3. Language acquisition—Parent participation. 4. Interpersonal communication in infants. I. Title.
  BF720.C65C334 2015
  419'.1—dc23

                          2014048802

          Printed and bound in the United States of America.

              VP 10 9 8 7 6 5 4 3 2 1

CONTENTS

Chapter Four: Let's Communicate! Thirteen
to Eighteen Months

Your baby is primed for communication and is motivated by all
the new things he is learning. These easy strategies will develop
these abilities to help you both communicate better.

Chapter Five: I Can Talk and Sign! Nineteen
to Twenty-Four Months

Your baby is transitioning from signing to talking, but signing
can still benefit your baby even after she can speak, including
increasing her vocabulary.

Chapter Six: Now What? Two Years and Beyond

If your toddler is not speaking yet, signing will keep the
communication going until he is ready. If your toddler is
speaking, you can use his signing abilities to facilitate
future learning.

PREFACE

PARENTS HAVE ALWAYS STRUGGLED TO communicate with their babies in the early months and years. Usually, parents do all the talking and babies most of the listening, with some interaction through grunts, looks, sounds, and gestures that parents try to interpret. This mostly one-way communication was better than nothing, but it still caused a lot of frustration and confusion for both.

THE GOOD NEWS

The secrets of how to create two-way conversations with your baby at an earlier age are easily accessible! By using basic signs with your baby—also called baby sign language—you can begin the conversation much earlier. This book will teach you exactly how to do that by using your child's natural learning tendencies to create two-way conversations.

Baby Signing Essentials is designed as a great resource for age-specific guidance on what to do at each age so that you can get started signing with your baby today. Since there is a great difference between a four-month-old and a twelve-month-old, each chapter provides a brief overview of what is going on developmentally with your baby during a specific age and then teaches you the most important signs at that age. Baby sign language is not rocket science, but knowing a few good tricks and tips makes it easier. Remember, keep things simple and follow the easy-to-accomplish steps for the greatest success.

HOW IT WORKS

This book can be approached in two ways. It's designed chronologically so that you can read it from cover to cover to get a complete idea of your child's progression and what works best at each age to facilitate successful communication. Or, if you are a busy mom or dad who needs a quick and easy overview of the basics, you can flip to the chapter that corresponds to your baby's age and dive in.

Beginning with chapter 2, each chapter also includes the following helpful resources:

* So What's Happening Now?: This section describes your baby's development, so you know exactly what to expect as your baby grows.
* All You Need: This section right before the signs in each chapter gives you a quick list of the most important signing instructions and ideas to do with your baby at each age.
* Essential Signs: At the end of each chapter is a list of ten or fifteen essential signs for each age so you know which ones to start with. You can always learn more of the signs included in each chapter, but these are the ones that have proven most useful. If you are looking for a specific sign, there is an alphabetical listing of all signs on page 197.

Note: When you see words that are bolded and in capital letters (**APPLE** or **MORE**), these are the words that you will sign with your baby.

Note on gender: As you read through the book, you may notice it alternates between gender references in each section. This is to give babies of both genders equal focus and avoid unnecessary or confusing repetition. This book is for all babies and their parents.

Parenting is an amazing experience, and signing with your child can really enhance the journey for both of you. This book will help you understand ways to gain more joy and insight into each other, and I hope it will help you build a strong foundation of great communication and love that will last you the rest of your lives.

ACKNOWLEDGMENTS

BEING A MOTHER IS A great journey that teaches you a lot. Without my two children, I never would have embarked on the baby sign language journey. The moms who shared their stories to enrich this book feel the same way. Thank you to them for sharing their experiences. Thanks to Dr. Joseph Garcia and his generous and loving soul. Without his vision for using American Sign Language (ASL) with babies, my relationship with my children would be less fulfilling. Thank you to Tricia Taylor for inspiring me to take my homemade flash cards and turn them into a product, lessons, classes, books, and more. Thank you to Shelly Parcell and Henry, who renewed my love for signing with babies through our friendship and watching Henry communicate his amazing thoughts.

Thank you to my mother, who gave me life and told me I could do anything. You continue to encourage me. Thank you to my best friend and husband, who supports me in everything and almost never says no, even when he doesn't understand my journey. Our life is an adventure. Thanks to God for the opportunities that have made it possible for me to learn and sign with my own babies. My life with my children wouldn't be as rich without baby sign language. And thank you to the two precious souls who enliven my life every day. Seeing the world through their eyes makes the world a much better place.

CHAPTER ONE

START THE ADVENTURE!

BABY SIGN LANGUAGE HAS BEEN featured everywhere from the news to the movies. But if you're picking up this book, it's likely you want to know more about it than these sound bites and clips offer. You may be wondering whether there is an official "language" called baby sign language and what exactly it means and when to use it. Or you may want to be able to communicate with your baby better but worry that if you sign with your child, she might not talk.

This chapter takes a look at what baby sign language is, its origin, why it works, and what myths might be out there about it. It explains what it can do for you and for your baby, as well as what it won't do.

WHAT IS BABY SIGN LANGUAGE?

We all use language to understand what is said to us (*receptive language*) and to express ourselves (*expressive language*). *Language* is how we communicate with others using words, signs, or writing. Language includes the types of words we use (nouns, verbs, adjectives, adverbs), how many words we use, how we put the words together to form thoughts, and so on. *Speech* is how we pronounce words and show the language we have acquired.

Believe it or not, before babies can speak, they have a language of their own, communicating with others by using grunts, visual cues, and gestures. Babies naturally point at things they want, wave with their hands to say good-bye, and clap to show excitement. These are all signs. Baby sign language taps into these natural tendencies to gesture with their hands to communicate their needs, wants, and even complex thoughts. You just teach them simple signs for things they want, and they use those to explain to you what they need. It takes a little patience and dedication on Mom and Dad's part, but any baby can do it. And the best part is that it fits right into your daily routine. Just add signs to the conversations and communications you already have with your baby.

Think about how empowering this can be for your baby. Instead of crying and hoping you can guess that she needs her diaper changed or wants to have some applesauce, she can tell you. You don't have to be standing in the grocery store line with a screaming baby wondering whether she is hungry or tired or bored. She can let you know. Baby sign language has the power to stop tantrums and start conversations and create a closer bond with your child.

BENEFITS OF SIGNING WITH YOUR HEARING BABY

Hearing babies who sign with their parents and other caregivers have a unique opportunity to learn to communicate their needs and wants and thoughts long before the average hearing child can. Signing has short-term benefits—reduced frustration and the ability to communicate—that are really important. But it also has long-term benefits—increased vocabulary, IQ, and interest in reading—that will help your child as he grows and matures. What you are doing now will help lay an important foundation for your child's educational mind-set. Signing will help him enjoy learning and develop the necessary skills to learn well.

In addition to the benefits for your child, signing with your baby will help you have a more enjoyable relationship with your child. You will be less stressed out and will be able to understand his specific needs instead of guessing what that cry at 3:00 a.m. means. As your baby grows, you will have less of the "terrible twos" to deal with than other parents. This is because most of these tantrums come from your baby's inability to specifically tell you what he needs. Without this skill, he is left with what he knows—crying. And fewer tantrums are never a bad thing.

A final thing to consider is that even if you are already in tune with your baby, using baby sign language allows your baby to communicate his needs to others who don't have your sixth sense for his needs but who have learned a few basic signs. That is very important for making your baby independent.

BABIES WHO SIGN

* Speak at the normal time or sooner.
* Have larger vocabularies.
* Have more interest in reading.
* Have better skills in spelling and reading.
* Score higher on verbal and language tests.
* Have higher IQ scores at age eight (see Table 1).
* Have more self-confidence because they get their needs met.
* Have a start on a second language.
* Develop both sides of their brains at a higher rate.
* Have an easier time transitioning between languages in a bilingual house.
* Have parents who are less frustrated by trying to guess needs.
* Have a close bond with their parents.

WHEN WILL YOUR BABY BEGIN TO SPEAK?

For those of you who are worried that signing with your baby will cause her to start talking later in life (or not at all), fear not! Longitudinal research funded by the National Institutes of Health studied signing children for an extended period of time and found the children who signed spoke sooner than their counterparts who did not sign. Regardless of whether or not you sign with your baby, speaking is one of the last skills your baby will master in her early communicative development because it is one of the most complex skills to learn. She must learn to control and maneuver the muscles in her tongue, cheeks, and lips, as well as control her breathing, all while directing airflow to make a noise. In contrast, your baby has enough control over her hands to make a basic sign somewhere between four and eight months and to make more complex signs somewhere between seven and twelve months. The NIH's research found that during the time they could not speak, the signing children could communicate. When they began to speak, they had larger vocabularies, learned new words faster, and spoke in more complex sentences (see Table 1).

Your baby will probably speak sooner if you sign, because when you do, you are not actually being silent. You are speaking directly to her. She can see your mouth, hear your voice, and see the sign. In fact, she is getting more linguistic input than most babies. Parents often talk to their babies with their backs turned, while they are on the phone, or while the child is distracted. None of these are optimal situations for learning to speak. When you sign with your baby, you look at her and she looks at you. You won't be distracted, and she will see and hear you speak, which helps her learn to communicate.

Additionally, you are engaging your baby in a conversation at a much earlier age. Because you expect her to respond when she can, you are inviting her into the conversation. Once she begins signing, she can initiate and direct your conversations. As she feels more empowered, your baby also realizes that speaking gives her even more ability to communicate with you and gives her what she needs more quickly.

Babies who sign make their first sentences (two or more words together) up to six months earlier than babies who do not sign—as early as twelve to fourteen months of age—and they will make three-word sentences up to a year earlier than babies who do not sign. The average child who does not sign makes his first two-word sentence somewhere between eighteen and twenty-four months and three-word sentences somewhere close to three years old.

TABLE 1
Verbal Abilities of Children Who Don't Sign versus Children Who Do Sign

Age	Developmental Norm	Signing Children
12 months	Possible 2–3 spoken words	25 signs/16 spoken words
18 months	6–15 spoken words	79 signs/105 spoken words with some sentence development using both words and signs
24 months	50 spoken words/2–3-word sentences with a vocabulary of 150–300 words	Speech like 27–28-month-old (200–300 words)/3–5-word sentences with a vocabulary of 200–500 words
36 months	Understands 800 words/Uses 3–5-word sentences easily	Speech like 47-month-old (up to 1500 words)/almost total control of everyday language
8 years	IQ Score of 102 for control group	IQ Score of 114 for signing group

Sources: Steven P. Shelov, ed., *Caring for Your Baby and Young Child: Birth to Age 5*, 5th ed. (New York: Bantam, 2009); "Speech and Language Development Milestones," MayoClinic.com; M. E. Anthony and R. Lindert, *Signing Smart with Babies and Toddlers* (New York: St. Martins Griffin, 2005); S. Goodwyn, L. Acredolo, and C. Brown, "Impact Of Symbolic Gesturing on Early Language Development," *Journal of Non-Verbal Behavior* 24 (2000): 81–103; L. Nicolosi, E. Harryman, and J. Kresheck, *Terminology of Communication Disorders: Speech-Language-Hearing*, 5th ed. (Philadelphia: Lippincott Williams & Wilkins, 2003); L. Acredolo and S. W. Goodwyn, "The Long-Term Impact of Symbolic Gesturing During Infancy on IQ At Age 8," paper presented at the meetings of the International Society for Infant Studies, Brighton, UK (July 2000).

At the age of two years, most babies can say somewhere around fifty words, generally with one or two syllables each. They can put a few two-word or three-word sentences together, such as "I want milk" or "Give ball." When my son was twenty-two months old, he spoke hundreds of words and used complex sentences. I remember one in particular because he used a word I had not taught him. We had been having issues with our car and had told him that the car would be fixed at the "car doctor." One day, he looked in the garage and noticed the car was missing. He turned around and looked at me and said the following words exactly: "Did Daddy take the car to the dealership?" Think about what he said. He used an eight-word sentence with past tense and a huge word—dealership. He must have heard us talking about the dealership and made the connection in his head that this is what the "car doctor" was. After I recovered from my amazement, I answered yes, the car was at the dealership.

The research shows that no delay in spoken language acquisition occurs in children who sign. Ignore anyone who claims your child will become mute, deaf, or both because you are signing. (None of this will happen!) You are doing an amazing thing for your child, possibly even more amazing than you think.

A VERY IMPORTANT TIME FOR LEARNING

In the first three years of life, a baby's brain grows and develops more significantly than at any other time. This is when a baby learns how to think, respond, and solve problems, and a baby's brain is twice as active as the average adult's brain during these years. These first three years are a very special opportunity for parents. They are a crucial time for learning, because babies have the greatest potential to soak up and retain information.

While genetics are important and do influence what skills and abilities your child will have, new research shows that environment plays an equally important role in early development. Neuroscientists are now finding that early experiences impact a baby's brain development greatly. This means that

The Zero to Three website is a great resource to help you know what your baby should be doing during the first three years of life. www.zerotothree.org.

you have an incredible chance to have a positive impact that will help develop his potential.

To illustrate my point further, here's an example: A friend of mine wanted to sign with her son after seeing my son's success. But she felt that our results were mostly due to the fact that my son was what she called "really smart"— that he was just naturally advanced. I disagreed with her and asked her to sign with her son and see what happened. To her surprise (but not mine), her son followed almost exactly the same linguistic learning pattern that my son did—nurture at work. He learned to communicate using signs, began to speak words at around fourteen months, learned the alphabet on his own at around eighteen months, was speaking clearly in two- to three-word sentences by twenty months, and was linguistically advanced at his second birthday. He has also developed the same interest in math that my son has, and he is learning to read at three years old (the same age at which my son got interested in reading). His speech is so good that he corrects his parents when they make grammatical errors—and that makes us all smile.

ANOTHER REASON WHY SIGNING WORKS SO WELL

Signing with your baby helps your child develop more than just an ability to communicate. Parents have noted that their children who sign tend to be well adjusted, more even tempered, more polite, and generally better learners as well. Why? Scientists have shown that certain factors in the first years can help children develop to their full potential. According to the American Academy of Pediatrics (AAP), these include the following:

* Feeling special and valued
* Feeling safe and loved
* Knowing what to expect from their environment
* Having guidance

* Experiencing a balance of freedom and limits
* Being exposed to language (and to more than one if possible)
* Being exposed to play, exploration, books, music, and age-appropriate toys

Using sign language with your baby will help you do all of these things. The environment you create for your child really does affect him, and when you use sign language, you are given extra tools to help facilitate learning and growth in your baby.

By interacting with your child in the earliest stages, you can develop communication and language skills, identify developmental problems earlier, create a stimulating environment, and have a positive parenting experience. Your relationship becomes a two-way interaction. Amazing!

SO WHEN CAN WE START?

By the age of four months, your baby goes from being a newborn—totally dependent on you—to a baby who can control more of her responses. She'll also start interacting with you. So starting to sign sometime between four and six months is a great time. When you notice that your baby holds your gaze and watches what you do, she is ready for you to start signing.

However, communication doesn't have to wait until your baby is ready to sign. Even during the first three months, babies are very receptive to your talking them through daily activities. Babies differentiate sounds very early and can figure out how words begin and end. They can also distinguish different inflections as early as six months.

As you are nursing or feeding, have a conversation with your baby. When you go to bathe your baby, tell her you are going to give her a bath. You can even describe the process you are going through as you do it. "Sadie, we are going to take a bath now. See, here is your bathtub. The water is warm and the soap smells good. Do you like having your head scrubbed? Now we are going to rinse you off and take you out of the tub. Doesn't this dry, warm towel feel nice?" You get the picture.

You can vary your conversations by singing and reading books to your baby. You can sing your favorite top-ten songs or children's songs. If you speak with your baby during the day for the first three months, you are getting yourself in the habit of creating communication opportunities. Then, when your baby is ready to see you sign at about four months old, you are already in a communication routine. All you need to do is add signs to your conversations.

WHAT IF MY BABY WILL BE CARED FOR BY SOMEONE ELSE?

Many parents return to the workforce and are worried about how a caregiver will react to the idea of signing with your baby. If your baby's primary caregiver is older, you might hear things like, "In our day, we never signed with babies and we got along just fine." Or if the caregiver has more than one child to take care of, she might feel she doesn't have time to learn signs.

There are a few ways to approach the situation with your caregiver. You could give her this book and ask her to read it. She may become convinced after reading it that signing has made a difference in the lives of other families. You can show her clips on signing from the Internet. If you have friends who have signed with their children, ask them to talk to her about their personal experience or let her watch their interactions with their child.

A caregiver's reluctance to sign with your baby may stem from fears that she has to learn a whole new language to sign with your child. Alleviating these fears may solve your problem. You can even limit the number of signs your caregiver will use to as few as five to ten signs. Even a few signs will help both your baby and his caregiver. This approach often also works well with fathers who are reluctant to sign or grandparents who think this is just a fad.

If your attempts to persuade your child's primary caregiver to sign with your baby fail, you can still be successful in signing with him. Just sign when you are together. It may take more time for your baby to sign back, but when he does communicate using signs, often caregivers give in and learn a few signs.

Lauri had to return to work soon after her daughter Alexa was born. She entrusted the care of her daughter to her mother-in-law for several hours a day. Lauri began signing with Alexa when she was six months old and discussed this with her mother-in-law, who immediately refused to sign with her granddaughter. At first, Lauri was disappointed but decided to keep signing when she was with Alexa. "It was hard because we did not have a lot of time together, and I felt like Alexa was not seeing enough signs for it to matter. Her grandmother would not sign with her at all. It took Alexa longer to sign back, but when she was about twelve months old, she began signing with me. Her first sign was **MORE**. She wanted more cereal. I was so shocked when I saw her sign the first time.

"Over the next few months, she began to sign more often and use more signs. She would also sign to her grandmother, but her grandmother didn't know what she was doing. One day, my mother-in-law asked why Alexa tapped her fingers together. When I told her that meant she wanted more of something, my mother-in-law was amazed. Since then, she has learned three or four signs that help her with Alexa. She won't learn more than that, but Alexa and I are fine with it. We still sign at home, and Alexa now knows about twenty-five signs."

BUT WILL MY BABY SIGN?

Many parents are concerned that their baby will not sign. As long as your baby does not have any disabilities or developmental setbacks, his success in signing will have more to do with your willingness to teach him than with anything else. If you are consistent in your signing interactions, your baby should catch on and sign back when he has the motor skills to do so. Until he has the motor skills, he may respond through grunts or gestures, so keep that in mind.

EXPERIENCES OF SIGNING FAMILIES

Hundreds of thousands of families have signed with their babies. Some have learned as few as three signs and found that to be effective for them. Most families have learned somewhere between twenty and fifty signs. This book is designed to help you do this easily. But others go on to learn many more signs. Here are a few stories from families who are signing with their children.

Jennifer and Alice

Jennifer started signing with her daughter Alice at seven months. She started with **DOG**, **MILK**, **EAT**, and **MORE**. Jennifer first noticed that Alice would nod her head and make grunting noises at about eight or nine months when Jennifer signed **MILK**. Alice made her first sign (**DOG**) at ten months. It took Alice only a month longer to feel comfortable with signing. At fourteen months, she now understands about one hundred signs and signs using about fifty signs.

Jennifer says, "We were at the pool this summer, and my daughter Alice had just started signing **BABY**. I wasn't sure what she was doing, because she had just started using that sign a few days prior. I said, '**BABY**?' and looked around. Sure enough, about fifty feet away, there was a mother nursing her baby. My daughter always looks so pleased when she's made a connection. It's beautiful." Another time, Jennifer and Alice were shopping when Alice began to sign **MILK**. "I was in the middle of a conversation with a friend (a new father himself), but I didn't skip a beat and handed her the milk. My friend said, 'How did you know what she wanted?' I replied that she had told me and showed him the sign. He just looked shocked." Jennifer says that everyone in the family signs with Alice and this "encourages her to continue learning. Seeing into the window of the baby's mind is amazing!"

Lauri, Megan, and Max

Lauri signs with both her children, Megan and Max. She relates the following about her daughter: "Megan was eleven months when she was sitting in her doll's crib. I told her to come out (I didn't want her to break it), but she insisted. Then I said to her 'It's for your baby doll.' Then she looked at me and shook her head and signed boat. She was pretending it was a boat. At her young age, she was *pretending*, and I was able to play with her instead of ruining it for her. I got a box and we continued to play boat." Being able to sign with Megan gave Lauri a way to understand what her daughter was really doing and let her respond in a way that gave both of them what they needed.

Lauri's son Max also benefits from signing. When Max was twelve months old, Lauri had the following experience: "Max was trying to get a lid off a jar. He looked at me and signed **HELP** and showed me the jar. I asked what he wanted with it; he signed hat and then pointed to the lid. He was able to use the limited signs he knew to get his point across that he wanted the lid off the jar. Using the sign hat let him communicate with me instead of throwing the jar at me in a fit (his usual reaction of frustration)."

Thalia, Lance, and Trinity

Thalia is a mother to twenty-month-old twins, Lance and Trinity. Twins tend to talk late because they can create their own "language" to communicate with each other. Also, because there are two babies, people tend to talk to both of them rather than directly to one or the other. Thalia says, "It was my hope that teaching them to sign would allow them to communicate with me sooner and that I wouldn't have to wait for them to begin verbal communication to understand what they were saying. I first began signing with them at six months. I started with **MORE**, **CHANGE DIAPER**, and **EAT**. After a couple of months, I gave up. When I started back up again around the middle of their eleventh month, I added **ALL DONE**, **MOM**, and **DAD**.

"Trinity began to pick it up immediately. It was almost as if something had been unlocked for her. She signed back within a few weeks. She signed **MORE** and then **ALL DONE** followed the very next day. Once she started signing, she just couldn't be stopped. Now she understands hundreds of signs, and she signs using one hundred to one hundred thirty signs. Lance liked signing immediately as well, but he had no desire to sign back to me until he signed **AIRPLANE** at fourteen months old. Anytime he saw or heard an airplane, he was quick to make that sign. He also signed **AIRPLANE** when he saw helicopters, leaf blowers, and lawn mowers. He didn't sign anything else until he was sixteen months old, but he signed **AIRPLANE** a lot. Now Lance recognizes probably one hundred signs, but he signs only around fifty to seventy signs."

Kim and Gage

Kim, who is a speech-language pathologist, began signing with her younger son, Gage, when he was about eight months old. "Our first family picture shows him approximating the sign for **MORE** (he was about nine months old) because the photographer was using a squeaky puppet to make the boys smile. When Gage was about twenty-two months old, he hadn't yet progressed to using words. I had been worried for a while, but all my family and friends kept telling me to wait and said, 'You know too much; you are too close to it.' Our older son talked late, but he began with sentences. He went from no words to more than fifty words and phrases between fifteen and eighteen months. He continued to talk above expectation. Gage was the second child, with an older brother who did stuff for him and wouldn't shut up, so I decided to wait a bit longer. He babbled loads and used more than three hundred signs, even three- to four-word phrases, so I decided to have him evaluated by a colleague.

"I thought he might have a problem with the muscles in his mouth. Sure enough, my fears were confirmed and he was diagnosed as apraxic (a motor coordination disorder that affects speech skills). Gage remained unintelligible for another six or so months. At about two and a half years, he got to the point where some people, other than me, his dad, and my mom, could understand him. Even though through the whole process he couldn't use words to tell us what he wanted or needed, he did sign. I can't imagine how we would have gotten through it without sign. You just never know when it will be 'a neat thing to do' versus a tool that will be needed for a child's development. We still sign today for literacy, reading skills, behavior management, and songs—and we all love it."

ALL YOU NEED (BIRTH TO FOUR MONTHS)

- Baby sign language is simple and builds on your baby's natural tendency to gesture and his desire to communicate to help him communicate early.
- The first three years of life are the most important develop-mental time in your baby's life, so use them wisely to teach great learning patterns.
- Your baby will be ready to sign at four months (next chapter), but start talking with your baby from birth to help her learn the rules of language by talking, singing, and reading.
- If your baby will be cared for by someone else, discuss your desire to sign with your baby and explain how it can help your caregiver and your baby bond and communicate.

CHAPTER TWO

SHOW ME!—FOUR TO SEVEN MONTHS

AT FOUR MONTHS, YOUR BABY is ready for you to start signing. He can now see you across the room, and when you talk to him, he probably coos and smiles. He is watching how you communicate and is learning the subtle rules of language. Even though it may be several months until your baby signs back to you, he is ready to have you add signs to your conversations. Most babies sign back somewhere between seven and ten months, but before then, they will respond to your signs in other ways that let you know the message is coming through loud and clear.

In this chapter, we'll take a look at the following:

* ❋ How your baby is developing from four to seven months
* ❋ How to start signing with your baby
* ❋ What signs to start signing with your baby

You know your baby better than anyone. Take things at her pace. If she was premature, you might need to adjust everything to her gestation date and expect that she may not sign as soon as other babies. Or if she has another developmental issue, you might need to adapt things even more.

SO WHAT'S HAPPENING NOW?

Right now your baby is learning to coordinate his senses of touch, vision, and hearing. His motor skills are increasing as well. He is learning to grasp, roll over, sit up, and may even be crawling by the end of this period.

In addition to the increases in sensory and physical coordination, your baby now has more ability to choose his own actions and reactions. He will learn to pick up and explore a toy, or he may cry because he wants to change activities. He will become more interactive and might become a show-off, smiling and playing with anyone. This is the period when your baby's personality really begins to blossom. It is also a key time to start signing with your baby. Because your baby is becoming more alert and more interested in the world around him, he is primed for watching and learning from you.

Every day with your baby will be a new adventure as he gains new skills and explores his personality. Even if this is not your first child, your relationship will be different because this baby is different. Signing will help you learn more about your baby and see into his thoughts and personality. So embrace this exciting reality and enjoy the experience.

Motor Development

During this period, your baby gains greater control over her body. She is learning to sit up, roll over, and use her hands to grasp. Your baby does not have the manual dexterity to make very many signs at this age and may not have the control to make distinctive signs until she is seven to nine months old. But it is not uncommon for parents who start to sign with their babies around four months to see their babies attempt to make a sign back. Generally, babies will sign **MILK** or **MORE** as their first sign.

If your baby does not attempt to sign, don't worry. Babies who can't yet get their hands together to sign will respond in other ways—some even very amusing. My son, for example, panted when I asked him if he wanted milk or when I made the sign for **MILK**. A friend's son squealed in delight when his mother would sign **MILK**.

Visual Development

Your baby's eyesight is also improving and will continue to develop until about seven months. Now, he can see clearly several feet in front of his eyes and can track faster and faster movements. He can follow a ball as it rolls across the room, is stimulated by a mobile, and enjoys more complex patterns and movements. Adding signing to the conversation you have had with your baby since birth adds visual interest to your interactions and will engage your baby further in your communications.

Language Development

This is a great time of language development for your baby. She begins to distinguish individual sounds and how these sounds combine into words and sentences. Your baby can recognize her name. When you call to her, she will turn her head toward you. She will also recognize the names of the people she associates with most—mommy, daddy, brother or sister, etc.

Your baby will also start to babble during this time. Listen closely to your baby's babbling, and you will recognize that she is working out linguistic characteristics. She will raise and drop her voice as if she is asking a question or making a statement. You can reinforce this by picking up on the sounds your baby is working on and building on the conversation with both sounds and signs. If your baby is making the sound "mah," you can sign and say "You sound like you are saying **MOM** [make the sign when you say it]. I am so glad you want to say **MOM**. Mom, mom."

Cognitive Development

Your baby's cognitive abilities are growing by leaps and bounds. His attention span and memory are increasing. He is learning the concept of cause and effect and will undoubtedly spend a lot of time experimenting with this (i.e., the dreaded drop-a-spoon-so-mom-picks-it-up cause-and-effect experiment). By the end of seven months, your baby will also begin to understand that things exist even when he cannot see them, which is why your baby cries when you leave the room (more on that in chapter 3). This is called *object permanence*. Your baby's understanding that things exist that he cannot see will also help him to find partially hidden objects. This is a good time to start playing peekaboo or hiding games.

> It is increasingly important to engage your baby in linguistic learning from six to nine months, as this is when your baby actively imitates the sounds of speech. The American Academy of Pediatrics suggests that some of the best words to introduce your baby to at four to seven months are simple words such as:
>
> * baby   * milk
> * cat   * eat
> * dog   * walk
> * go   * mama
> * hot   * dad
> * cold

Social Development

At the beginning of this period, your baby may seem very passive, but toward the end, she may become much more assertive—showing the stuff she is really made of. As she gains more physical and cognitive abilities, she becomes more eager to reach out and interact with the world around her, especially with you and other caregivers. She may become a bit more demanding of your attention, as you are the best teacher and audience she has. This makes the period starting at about six months a stellar time to sign with your baby.

Your baby enjoys social play and responding to others—excellent conditions for introducing more signs.

LET'S GET SIGNING!

If you are excited to start, go ahead and start right around four months. Starting around six months is also generally a great time, since babies begin to do things such as play, eat, and move, and you will have more topics to "discuss." Think of all the things you will be able to sign with your baby as he learns to eat: "Do you want to **EAT**? Yum. I have some **BANANA** for you. Do you want **MORE BANANA**? OK. We are **ALL DONE** with the **BANANA**. Do you want some **MILK**?"

Start Simple

Now you are ready to start signing with your baby! It's best to start with five to ten signs. Choose a few signs for things you need and a few signs for things your baby is interested in. To make it easier for you to remember the signs and incorporate them into what you do, think about them in relation to the activities in which you will be using them. Some of the signs that are best to start with are listed below by activity, and many of these can be used in more than one situation.

MEAL SIGNS

* MILK
* MORE
* EAT
* ALL DONE/FINISHED

DIAPER/DRESSING SIGNS

* CHANGE DIAPERS
* ALL DONE
* LIGHT or FAN

ACTIVITY SIGNS

* BOOK
* ALL DONE/FINISHED
* MORE
* PLAY
* MUSIC

BATH SIGNS

* BATH
* ALL DONE/FINISHED

BEDTIME SIGNS

* BOOK
* MUSIC
* SLEEP or BED

These signs are effective because:

* They are distinct. Each sign looks different than the other signs, so there is no way to confuse them.

* They relate to the things your baby is doing.
* They can be used in situations that occur often during the day.

Keep in mind that whether you choose five or ten signs to start with is not as important as choosing signs that interest your baby and that you will use often.

THE SUPER SEVEN SIGNS

IF YOU DON'T LEARN ANY OTHER SIGNS, LEARN THESE:

1. MILK
2. MORE
3. EAT
4. CHANGE DIAPERS
5. BATH
6. ALL DONE/FINISHED
7. BOOK

Sign in Context

You never need to make a specific time for signing. Just incorporate signing into whatever you are doing with your baby. Show the sign while you are interacting with the concept or object. For example, you can sign **MILK** while feeding your baby a bottle or while nursing. Or, if your baby is eating solids, sign **EAT** while your baby eats. Remember that babies live in the here and now. If you say "We are going to read a **BOOK**," make sure you are ready to do it now. Your baby won't understand that he has to wait for it.

HOW TO SIGN WITH YOUR CHILD

Talking helps your baby develop an understanding of language. Always speak with your child when you are signing. Speak in complete sentences even though you may be using only one or two signs for the entire sentence. If you say "Do you want some **MILK**?" you will only sign **MILK** for the entire sentence you are speaking.

Whenever you sign and speak, talk directly to your child. Speak clearly as you sign and give added vocal emphasis to the word you are signing. When you ask "Do you want some **MILK**?" accentuate the word "milk" and repeat the sign several times. This exaggerated signing allows your baby to see the sign you are making and associate it with the situation.

Have conversations with your baby about what you are doing. When she is nursing or drinking a bottle, say "I bet you are enjoying your **MILK**. It is good **MILK**. You are so cute when you drink your **MILK**." This might seem funny to us as adults, but it helps babies to hear the language and associate the words and signs with the activity.

Babies need to see things hundreds of times to learn. The key to success is using the signs as often as you can in meaningful events. Every time you eat, use the **EAT** sign, and repeat it frequently during the meal. Say "We're going to **EAT**. Do you want to **EAT**?" And then as you eat, say "Let's **EAT** another bite of cereal."

Engage Your Baby

One of the best ways to engage your baby is to intentionally focus on him. Make the sign directly in your child's line of sight so he can see your eyes, the sign, and your mouth. Then speak with your child, emphasizing the word you are signing. For example, you might say "Do you want some **MORE** apple?" Always speak directly to your baby. Get his attention. If you are far away, come closer to him. The act of coming closer lets him know that you are addressing him. If he is engaged in something else, use his name and touch him to get him to look at you. Vary your tone of voice so that it is not the same tone you use to speak on the

Parents who are successful with signing sign often. It is less important to know a lot of signs than to use the signs you know frequently. So if you find yourself having trouble remembering or being able to incorporate numerous signs into your interactions with your baby, again just focus on a few signs that you know you can use often.

phone. If you are talking about something that has sounds associated with it, you can even make those sounds to get his attention. For example, if you are feeding him, make eating noises or say "Yummy!" If you are talking about the family dog, bark.

Look for Baby's Response Back

You can tell your baby is looking to you for a sign when she looks at the object she wants you to sign (say, her toy) and then looks up at you, as if she is asking you for the sign. You will also know she is paying attention to your signs when she looks at your sign, then looks at her toy, and then looks back to you to see the sign again. Before she can make the sign, she will respond to you with a smile or giggles—especially if you guess what she wants and she gets it. Sometimes she will respond even without the conscious knowledge that she is doing it. Tricia began showing Keira the **MILK** sign at four months old. Then, about one and a half months later, Keira began to make the sign. At first Tricia was unsure that what she was seeing was a sign, because Keira would squeeze her fists as she nursed. But she realized that Keira did not squeeze her hands at any other time—just when she was nursing and had been shown the **MILK** sign.

Keep your eyes open—you may even see a sign this early. If not, don't be discouraged. As previously mentioned, most babies make their first sign between seven and twelve months, because this is when they have developed the manual dexterity to sign.

Involve the Family

If your baby interacts regularly with family members not in your immediate household (such as grandparents), now is a great time to introduce them to the idea of signing with your baby. Often, grandparents are amazed at the fact that they can communicate with their grandchildren at such an early age.

Pam is grandmother to Emily and several other grandchildren. She and her husband take care of four of their grandchildren daily in their home. When Pam's son and daughter-in-law decided to sign with Emily, Pam had not heard about signing with babies. She learned as Emily learned. "Emily would teach us. She signed **MILK, MORE, PLEASE, SHOES, SOCKS, COAT,** and more. It was really fun, and the three older cousins enjoyed it too. They learned the signs. Even though Emily is fifteen months younger than her cousins, we could understand her better. She could communicate with us." Pam says that Emily was milder and had fewer tantrums than her cousins. She talked ten months earlier than her cousins and had a larger vocabulary. "She is more confident that we know what she wants. And that is good for both of us."

A FINAL NOTE ON INCORPORATING SIGNS INTO LIFE

Sign whatever words you know as you speak with your baby. You might feel a bit strange having conversations with your baby before he can speak, but it is very important to do this, and you will soon find it enjoyable. You can incorporate signing into your reading time. Say and sign to him that you are going to read a book and then sign whatever pictures you know the signs for. Labeling the pictures in the story—telling what each object on the page is while pointing to it—helps to develop your baby's linguistic abilities.

Have a hard time remembering what to do or the signs to use? Copy the All You Need and Essential Signs sections in each chapter and paste them where you will use them.

ALL YOU NEED (FOUR TO SEVEN MONTHS)

Now is the time to start signing with your baby. Begin with just a few signs and then add more signs as your baby begins doing new things, such as playing and eating.

- Start with five to ten signs, choosing a few signs for things you need and a few signs for things your baby is interested in (see the Super Seven Signs).
- Incorporate signing into whatever you are doing.
- Show the sign while you are interacting with the concept or object.
- Speak in complete sentences even though you may only sign one sign.
- Talk directly to your child.
- Make the sign directly in your child's line of sight so he can see your eyes, the sign, and your mouth.
- Speak clearly as you sign and give added vocal emphasis to the word you are signing.
- Encourage any responses from your child, such as a small gesture or verbal engagement.
- Involve other family members.

SIGNS FOR FOUR TO SEVEN MONTHS

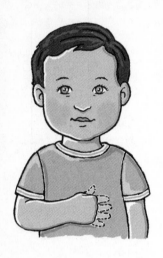

MILK

Squeeze like you are milking a cow.

Tip: Use for nursing or bottle-feeding. Parents get hung up on the delivery mechanism, breast or bottle—babies don't. When baby is hungry, ask "Do you want some **MILK**?" Have a conversation while feeding. "Yum. This **MILK** is so good." If you sign **MILK** out of context, you might need to feed him sooner.

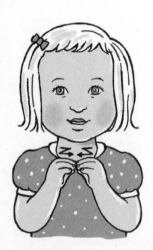

MORE

Tap fingers together.

Tip: This magical sign gives babies the power to get **MORE** of what they want. Introduce **MORE** at mealtime. Feed your baby a few bites of banana and then ask "Would you like some **MORE**?" Make the sign and then feed her more. As your interactions become more complex, you can even add two signs together and ask her "Do you want **MORE** to **EAT**?"

EAT/FOOD

Put food in your mouth.

Tip: At mealtime, say "Are you hungry? Do you want to **EAT**? Let's get you some **FOOD**." Later, you can learn the signs for specific foods such as banana, apple, cookie, cracker, and so forth.

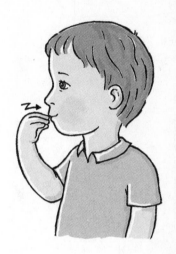

CHANGE DIAPERS

Rotate fists back and forth.

Tip: When babies learn that **CHANGE** means only a momentary stop in their play, they relax and allow their parents to change their diapers—especially useful when they are mobile.

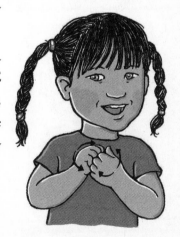

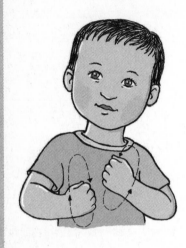

BATH

Scrub your chest.

Tip: Use as you get ready for a bath to get him in the right frame of mind. Keep both hands on your baby for now, but as he grows and can sit up on his own, then you can sign **BATH** during the bath.

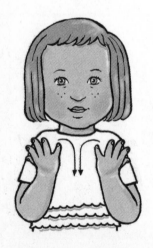

ALL DONE/FINISHED

Show that there is nothing in your hands.

Tip: Use to explain that you are finished doing one thing and are moving on to another. You can tell her that her bath is **ALL DONE**, or that you are **FINISHED** reading the book.

BOOK

Open and close a book.

Tip: Before you pick up a book and begin to read, say "We are going to read a **BOOK**. Let's choose a **BOOK** to read."

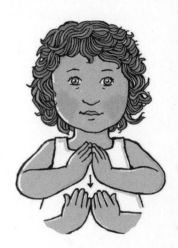

SLEEP

Pull hand across your face
to close your eyes.

Tip: Use when you get him ready for bed. He will eventually even be able to tell you when he needs to go to sleep.

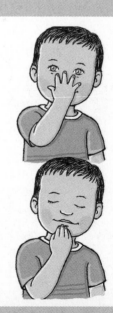

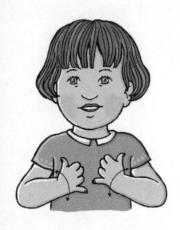

PLAY

Stick out your thumb and pinkie and swing your hands back and forth.

Tip: Use **PLAY** for tummy time and interacting on the floor. When older, **PLAY** helps your baby indicate that she wants to play with you. Babies can't make the sign for play well at first, so it will look like shaking fists or open hands until she can lift her thumb and pinkie finger.

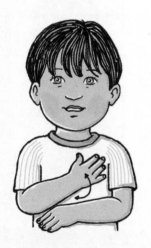

MUSIC/SING/SONG

Conduct music over your arm.

Tip: Use when you listen to music or sing. If you have a favorite song you sing to your baby, sign before you sing.

BED

Place hand on side of face like a pillow.

Tip: Some parents prefer to use this sign instead of **SLEEP**.

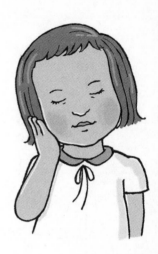

LIGHT

Open fingers to show
the light going on.

Tip: If your baby notices the lights when he is on the changing table, say "Yes, you are looking at the **LIGHT**. It is bright."

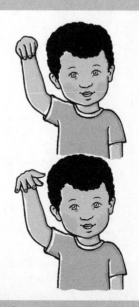

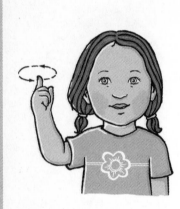

FAN

Move index finger around
in a circle above head.

Tip: Use if there is a ceiling fan where you change your baby.

ESSENTIAL SIGNS (FOUR TO SEVEN MONTHS)

Here are ten essential signs to learn and teach your baby at four to seven months:

1. MILK (see page 26)
2. MORE (see page 26)
3. EAT/FOOD (see page 27)
4. CHANGE DIAPERS (see page 27)
5. BATH (see page 28)
6. ALL DONE/FINISHED (see page 28)
7. BOOK (see page 29)
8. SLEEP (see page 29)
9. PLAY (see page 30)
10. MUSIC (see page 30)

CHAPTER THREE

WATCH ME!—EIGHT TO TWELVE MONTHS

FOR MOST BABIES, THE PERIOD from eight to twelve months is a time when they get mobile. Imagine what that must feel like. Finally a chance to get where you want to go! This is also the time when most babies make their first sign—even if you have been signing with them from birth. They now have the motor development to make signs, and if you have been signing with them for a few weeks or months, they have been primed for sign!

In this chapter, we'll take a look at the following:

* How your baby is developing from eight to twelve months
* What to expect from your baby's first signing attempts
* Strategies to increase your child's ability to sign
* Common questions and problems parents encounter
* Signs and activities to use in this period

SO WHAT'S HAPPENING NOW?

Your baby is a ball of constant motion. She is exploring her newfound abilities to sit up by herself, pick up things and examine them, and crawl or scoot on her bottom. She is now standing while holding onto the couch.

Just beginning now? If you haven't started signing with your baby yet, it's okay. You have not missed the window of opportunity. Just read the previous chapter and this chapter to get started.

She might even be ready to walk with the assistance of a table or couch. If she is really ready to move, she may be walking by the end of this period with little assistance.

Motor Development

While standing is a great milestone, your baby is also making great accomplishments in other areas of physical development that will aid his ability to sign. He is now learning to grasp objects with the pincer grasp—using his thumb and first or second finger. This means that your baby can make a wider variety of signs that were not physically possible for him before.

He is also learning to bang things together, another useful skill for signing words such as **MORE** and **BALL**. Many parents notice that their baby signs **MORE** by poking his index finger on the palm of his hand. This is very common. Don't worry about correcting his sign unless your baby is very receptive to your showing him how to sign it correctly. If you continue to sign it correctly while responding to his modification, he will change it over time on his own.

Language Development

Most babies whose parents have signed with them from four to seven months will start signing during this time. According to the American Academy of Pediatrics, even babies whose parents have not signed with them will now begin to point and gesture for things they want. Because you have been signing with your baby, her abilities will now begin to blossom, and you may even see an explosion of signs. (Hearing babies of deaf parents typically sign between fifty and one hundred signs by their first birthday because they see their parents signing so much.) If you use only ten to twenty signs, your relationship with your baby will still be better than if you didn't sign at all.

Your baby will also increase her verbal communications with you. Her earlier coos and gurgles will turn into more recognizable syllables such as "ba," "da," "ga," and "ma." She may even say words such as "bye-bye" or "mama." Her first syllables are not requests for something—rather she is practicing the sounds. But not everything is random at this age. She knows her name, and she can now understand when you sign and ask her questions such as "Do you want some **MILK**?" She may express her understanding with squeals or grunts or flailing arms, or she may even make the **MILK** sign back to you to say yes. She may become excited when you ask whether she wants to take a **BATH**. She understands more words and signs than you think.

Cognitive Development

At eight months, your baby is curious about everything around him. However, his attention span is actually about two to three minutes. Don't take it personally if you can't get through *Good Night Moon*. By twelve months, your baby may be more willing to sit through that if it's particularly interesting, but don't count on it.

Your baby is very interested in the details of things and interactions now. He will look at objects, feel textures, and experiment to discover the consequences of his actions. He will want to drop things off his high chair repeatedly to see what happens. You are part of his experiment. He will watch you intently to see what you do. This is one reason why most babies begin to sign in this period.

As he explores and experiments, he can become frustrated. Don't jump in too soon. Let your baby learn to handle small frustrations now so that he can handle greater frustrations in the future. Be available for him when he becomes too confused or upset, but stand back a bit and let him learn. Sometimes the most golden learning moments come when he is a bit frustrated and works the situation out on his own.

Social Development

This period is also a time for separation anxiety. Your baby may have easily gone to others before, but now she only wants you. This may even occur with the people she is around frequently, such as grandparents or caregivers. Your baby is reaching one of the first emotional milestones in her life. She is realizing that there is only one you—the first love of her life. She can now distinguish you from others, and she associates you with her well-being.

Separation anxiety also occurs because your baby now understands *object permanence*—the idea that something or someone still exists when she cannot see it or them. Don't be surprised if your baby soon begins to cry if you leave the room, as she now knows that you exist somewhere she is not. Generally, this reaction occurs sometime between the fourth and sixth month and intensifies through the tenth month.

Socially, your baby now has to learn about rules and limits. Because this is a time of new mobility, your baby is bound to get into things she shouldn't. She might need to learn not to touch certain objects at a relative's house or how to interact with the family dog. Often, distracting her is the best method to quickly solve the situation. If she is heading for the Ming vase, distract her and turn her attention toward the cuddly bear you are holding by changing your tone of voice to get her attention. Say something such as "Look at this wonderful **BEAR**. Does this **BEAR** look like fun to play with?" This often works better than saying no and expecting her to react. Her emotions and thought processes may not allow her to stop doing what she is headed for.

NOW THE SIGNING FUN BEGINS

Babies have the manual dexterity to make signs now, and they have the cognitive and social development to want to communicate their needs. When signing "clicks" with your baby, he will pick up signs more quickly. He may even begin to sign several different signs at once.

It may even seem that he is bursting with desire to communicate. He will look at you for

Learning not to do something she really wants to do is a major step toward learning self-control, and there will be times when your baby needs to know that something or someone is off limits. Babies who sign may have an easier time with limits, because they have a way to express these limits. Teaching your baby the signs for **STOP**, **NO**, and **HELP** will give her a way to understand what you expect of her. Keep your rules simple and stay consistent. But do not expect too much. Be patient and loving. Your baby still has very little sense of self-control.

the name and sign for everything he sees. Depending on how many signs you introduce, your baby will be able to recognize twenty to one hundred signs by his first birthday. He will make some of these signs, and some he may not be able to make yet. There are some signs that babies may never make. What busy baby who is on the move wants to make the sign for **WAIT**? He understands the concept and the sign when you make it, but he probably won't sign it back.

In addition to the signs he is learning, your baby may even have a vocabulary of two to four spoken words to go along with his signs—even if you are the only one who can understand him when he says them. If he doesn't say anything comprehensible, don't worry. Gibberish is good too.

Introduce Signs for Things Your Baby Sees

At this age, your baby understands that things have specific names. She will look to you to show her the names of everything in her world. This action is called *labeling*. Tell her what things are called, and if you know the sign for that thing, sign it too. Use the actual words for things and not made-up words—this will increase your baby's vocabulary. Your baby is better served by hearing the word "bottle" and seeing the sign for **MILK** than hearing you say "ba ba." If your baby says "ba ba" for her bottle, use the word "bottle" instead of repeating "ba ba," so that she hears and learns the correct word.

Make sure that you ask your baby questions about what she is looking at so that she can learn more. For example, when you are reading a book, say and sign "See the **BIRD**? Can you show me the **BIRD**?" She may be able point to it in the book and make the sign for it. This type of recognition shows that she knows the names and the signs for objects, and it will strengthen as she gets closer to her first birthday. If your baby is receptive when she is eight months old, take her hand and point it at the pictures in the book as you talk about them.

Increase Your Baby's Signing Abilities

There are several things you can do to help increase your baby's signing abilities.

Always do the following:

* Make sure that you get your baby's attention before you sign to him. Babies at this age are busy and on the move. Call his name, change your tone of voice, or touch your baby to get his attention.
* Make sure that you sign directly in your baby's line of sight. Make sure he can see your face and hands at the same time. This helps your baby to see your mouth, hear your voice, and see the sign.
* Make sure you and your baby are looking at the same thing. If he is looking at the bird and you are looking at the dog, he might get confused when you show him the sign for **DOG**.

When possible:

* Sign on your baby's body. Sometimes, it can be effective to get behind your baby and make the sign on his body or in front of his body. This helps your baby see what the sign looks like from the signer's perspective. For example, hold your baby on your lap and sign **EAT** right on his mouth.
* Help your baby make the sign. If your baby is receptive to having his hands manipulated, you can help him form the signs. Some children don't like to have their hands formed, so if your baby doesn't like this, don't worry.
* Point to the object you are signing. If your baby can see the object that you are signing about, point to the object so your baby will know what you are signing. This is especially effective when you are reading books and signing or when you are pointing out objects in your house such as food or toys.

By far, the most important key to increasing your baby's signing ability is to sign the signs you have chosen in as many situations as you can and as regularly as you can. If you are going to sign only five signs, use these signs often and in different situations. This will lead to more success than signing dozens of signs sporadically.

Sign as You Read

Reading to babies is a great way to encourage language development on several levels. When you read out loud, you introduce your child to the rich sound of language and the concept of words on a page. When you add signing to your reading experience, you make this process an interactive experience. Babies not only see the words and pictures and hear the sounds, but they also participate by signing along with you. Reading books becomes a fun and interesting experience for everyone.

Reading reinforces the concept that everything has a name and a sign. Choose books with simple stories and pictures of things relevant to your baby. Sign any words that you know. As your baby develops, books become even more important because they give her an opportunity to show you what she knows. Take a step back and let your baby lead the reading process. If she knows a few signs, let her express her knowledge by signing things she sees in the book. You can ask her questions about what she sees in the book and ask her to show you things. If she signs something, reinforce the sign with the spoken word for that sign: "Yes, that is a **BIRD!**"

GREAT BOOKS TO SIGN WITH

* *The Very Hungry Caterpillar* by Eric Carle: food signs
* *Brown Bear, Brown Bear* by Eric Carle: animal signs
* *The Going to Bed Book* by Sandra Boynton: bedtime and bath time signs
* *Curious George's Are You Curious?* by H. A. Rey: signs for emotions
* *Counting Kisses* by Karen Katz: signs for family members

Learn How to Read and Sign

It's hard to hold a book, sign, and keep track of a wiggly baby. But you can do it with a bit of practice and adaptation. Here are a few suggestions to try:

* If you and your partner are reading with your baby together, ask your partner to hold the book while you read and sign. This has the added dimension of showing your baby that reading is important to both parents. Switch and have your partner read and sign so that your baby has the chance to hear both voices read.

* If you are alone with your baby, put him on your lap and find a pillow to prop the book up. Then sign between the book and your baby's gaze.
* You can also hold the book with one hand and sign signs with the other hand. If you are reading an animal book while holding your baby, you can sign the animal signs on his body such as **ELEPHANT**, **GIRAFFE**, and so forth. Babies get a kick out of this, and it usually results in lots of giggles. If signs are made with two hands, use your baby as the "second hand," signing the signs on his body. For example, if you need to sign **BEAR**, tap one side of the **BEAR** sign on your baby's hand.

Don't stress out and get too worried about signing everything. Do what you can. Soon, you will be reading and your baby will be signing, so you won't need to be such an octopus.

Use Your Baby's Desire for MORE

As your baby learns about the world around her, she will want to repeat experiences and will use the sign **MORE** to help get what she wants. For your baby, **MORE** can mean "again," as in "Read that book **MORE** (again)." She will use **MORE** to indicate that she wants you to keep bouncing her. When you are playing, stop and ask her "Do you want **MORE** bounces?" Wait for her to respond with a sign or with a body movement or smile. Then continue. As she gets older, wait longer so that she can independently ask you for what she wants.

Mealtime is also a good time to use the sign **MORE**. You can say "Do you want some **MORE**? Let's have some **MORE CEREAL**." Then give your baby more cereal. Then wait a bit to give her the next bite. By having to wait, your baby might have the incentive she needs to make her first sign. Don't make your baby mad, but hesitate a bit and see whether she will ask you for more.

MORE is a very versatile sign and can help your baby express her desires to you. Use **MORE** when you are asking "Do you want to stay in the bath longer?" (**MORE BATH**). Or gather something that you have a lot of, such as balls, blocks, or stuffed animals, and play with them with your baby. Then hide them all from your baby's sight and then bring out one. Ask your baby whether she wants **MORE** blocks. Bring out another one and exaggerate your excitement. Keep going, asking whether she wants **MORE** each time and making each block's appearance an exciting event. Your baby will be entertained and will learn the concept of **MORE** in a different way. Then say "Wow, we have **A LOT** of blocks to play with!"

COMMON QUESTIONS AND CONCERNS ABOUT SIGNING

Invariably, in your signing experience, you will have a few moments when you have questions or concerns. Here are the most common situations and how to best approach them.

Your Baby Makes His Own Signs

You might find that your baby creates his own signs when he does not know a sign for something. This is a common step in the process of gaining language skills. Julie's fourteen-month-old son, Jake, makes his own signs. "He'll look me in the eye and start signing away, looking like a third-base baseball coach doing all kinds of meaningful gestures, but I have no idea what he's saying, because I don't know those signs! It's clear he's trying to tell me something, and that he's used to me understanding his gestures, and he doesn't quite get why I don't understand him when he does this. One of the most recent times he did this, he even repeated them more slowly, trying to get me to understand him. I have managed to figure out that when he points up in the air, he's saying 'outside,' so I'm learning."

Your baby may also be approximating a sign that is hard for him to make.

Sheia's twelve-month-old son, Kyler, signed **CRACKER** by knocking his fist on his head because he could not figure out how to knock his fist on his elbow. Once you figure out what your baby is signing, make sure that you validate his efforts to communicate with you. If there is an actual sign for the thing your baby is signing, show him the real sign and help him form it in his hand. If there's not a sign for that thing, you can accept your baby's made-up sign as a home sign and use it. This shows him that he is an integral player in the language process.

Your Baby Doesn't Sign Back

A few parents have come to me claiming that their baby just didn't like to sign. As we discussed the situation, I invariably found out that these parents were inconsistent in signing and could go for weeks without signing with their babies. No wonder their babies didn't sign back! Make sure that even if you sign only a few signs, you sign consistently, so that your baby learns that she can trust that you are willing to communicate with her.

Some parents don't give their baby time to sign back. Mom and Dad might be good at guessing what baby needs, but even though they sign to the baby, they don't wait to get the response back. If you say "Do you want some **MORE CEREAL**?" and then just give more cereal to your baby without waiting for her to respond, what reason does she have to sign back? Be patient. Sometimes the best learning comes when your baby wants something and realizes that if she wants it, she can ask for it. You don't need to get her frustrated, but the time between wanting something and getting it can be a golden moment for you to ask for a sign and wait for it. Give her a chance to respond to you.

If you have been consistent in signing and your baby has still not signed back, don't give up. Sometimes your baby will start signing only to stop or sign erratically. Don't worry. As babies develop, they are constantly learning, and sometimes signing takes a backseat to the other things they have on their minds, such as crawling or walking. Tammy shared the following: "I had been signing to my daughter since she was five months with no response. She is now almost eleven months, and just this past week, she mastered walking. She started signing the same week!" Keep signing and speaking, and your baby will continue to sign after she conquers the next milestone.

SIGNING AND ACTIVITIES FROM EIGHT TO TWELVE MONTHS

You and your baby can incorporate a lot of signs during the next eight to ten months. The following sections break down the signs that you may need to know at this age by the activities in which you will be using them.

Meal Signs

This period is a great time to introduce your baby to a wide variety of foods. Continue using the signs **MILK**, **MORE**, **EAT**, and **ALL DONE** that you were using previously. When you are ready to feed your baby, say "Do you want to **EAT**? Let's sit down and **EAT**." If you sign **EAT** every time you feed your baby, you introduce the sign for both **EAT** and **FOOD**, because they are the same sign.

Signing helps reduce the frustration babies feel as they begin to differentiate the foods they like and want. Carrie had been signing several different food signs with her son Nicholas. He had made a few signs back, but generally he signed **EAT** when he wanted food. One day, Carrie sat Nicholas down for lunch. She had fixed him a bowl of applesauce. Carrie knew he was hungry, but he would not eat the applesauce and started to get fussy. Carrie says, "I kept saying 'You love **APPLES**. Let's **EAT** some **APPLES**,' but he would not eat. Finally, he looked at me with a look that said, 'Mom you don't understand.' Then he signed **BANANA** and pointed to the bananas on the counter.

If he had not been able to sign, I would never have understood why he would not eat or what he wanted. We probably would have had a big crying session." Carrie quickly got Nicholas the banana he requested, and a crisis was averted.

Diaper/Dressing Signs

Your baby is getting more mobile and does not want to stop. This makes diapering a dicey situation. Just when you have your baby lying down with the diaper open and you are reaching for the wipes to clean off her poopy bottom, she decides it is time to get going. A few simple signs can help your baby understand that diapering won't last forever. You've already learned the sign **CHANGE**, and you are signing to your baby when you are going to change her diaper. If your baby tries to get up, you can say "You need to **WAIT**. I need to **CHANGE** your diaper." When you are finished, say "We are **ALL DONE!**"

Activity Signs

If your baby has a preference for a few toys, learn the signs for these toys. Some of the best signs to learn are **BALL**, **DOLL**, **CAR**, **TELEPHONE**, and **AIRPLANE**. You can play with the toys and say and sign them to your baby. Your baby is also ready to engage in games like peekaboo and hide-and-seek. Put a blanket over your head and ask "**WHERE** is **DADDY?**" Then let him pull the blanket off.

Safety Signs

One of the first signs you can show your baby is **NO TOUCH**. She will often be in situations where there are things that are off limits. You can only show this sign in context. When you see your baby going for something she should not touch, because it is dangerous or she could break it, remove her hand and get her attention and clearly explain "**DO NOT TOUCH** that." As your baby gets older, she might test the limits of what is a **NO TOUCH**. Make sure that you always react the same way, clearly and directly, that this is a **NO TOUCH** situation.

Bath Signs

Now that your baby is sitting up on his own in the bath, this becomes a wonderful place for him to play and explore. Let him splash in the tub and say "Yes, you can make the **WATER** move. Splash, splash goes the **WATER**." If he has toys in the bath, show him the signs for them, such as **BOAT**, **DUCK**, and **BALL**. You can say "Let's **PLAY** with your **BOAT**." However, don't be surprised if it is a while before he plays with the toys in the bath. Just the experience of being in the bath is a lot for your baby to take in.

Show your baby the signs for **WASH**, **WASH HAIR**, and **CLEAN**. He may really enjoy the process of getting clean, and you can enhance this by signing and singing while he is in the bath. The old song "The Mulberry Bush" can be changed to "Wash Our Baby." Make sure that when you are finished, you sign **ALL DONE** so that he knows the bath is over.

Bedtime Signs

Your baby needs to learn to fall asleep unassisted and put herself back to sleep if she wakes up. Sleep experts agree that having a nighttime ritual is one of the very best ways to prepare your baby for bed. You might read a **BOOK** or **SING** or give her a **BATH**. Doing these activities in the same order each night helps your baby prepare herself for the separation from you. You can also use the signs **ALL DONE** to help her understand that this is the end of your ritual and it's time for her to transition to **SLEEP**. In our house, we always read *The Going to Bed Book* right before going to bed. The book progresses through an evening ritual for getting ready for bed. We memorized the book, so when we would put our son to bed, we would quote the lines from the book that corresponded to the activity we were doing. That way, he could associate what he saw in the book with what he was experiencing.

A FINAL NOTE ON STAYING MOTIVATED

If you feel overwhelmed by signing, ask yourself if you are trying to "teach" your baby instead of just using signs with your daily

> Keep using the signs you started using with your baby from four to seven months. Add new signs that are of interest to your baby and help you communicate with each other. Don't feel like you have to be a super-parent. Just select a few at a time and take cues from your baby as to when to add more. You can always look ahead to the next chapter if you need more specific signs or look on page 197 for an alphabetical listing of all signs.

activities and conversations. If you are trying too hard, back off and just keep signing the basic signs you know. Then start adding signs when you feel comfortable again.

Sometimes babies stop signing because they are mastering another skill, not for lack of interest. If your baby is working on large motor skills such as crawling and walking and shows less interest in signing, just keep signing and he will begin to sign again when he has mastered his latest skill. You will both appreciate the ability to sign in the next several months, when his desire to express his independence and have his needs met grows exponentially.

ALL YOU NEED (EIGHT TO TWELVE MONTHS)

ALWAYS:
- Get your baby's attention before you sign to her.
- Sign directly in your baby's line of sight so she can see your face and hands at the same time.
- Make sure you and your baby are looking at the same thing.
- Look for signs your baby might make, even if they are just approximations of the sign, and encourage these first signs.
- Be consistent and patient—these are the keys to signing success.

WHEN POSSIBLE:
- Sign on your baby's body.
- Help your baby make the sign.
- Point to the object you are signing.

SIGNS FOR EIGHT TO TWELVE MONTHS
Food Signs

APPLE

Put knuckle of index finger
to cheek and twist it.

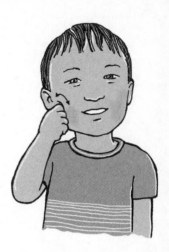

BANANA

Peel a banana.

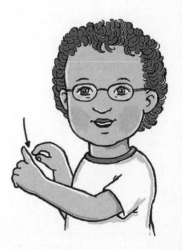

BREAD

Slice a loaf of bread.

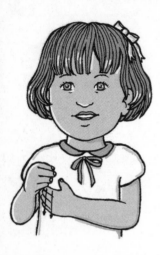

CEREAL

Wiggle finger across chin
like wiping off cereal.

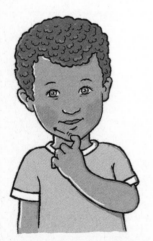

CHEESE

Press the cheese between hands.

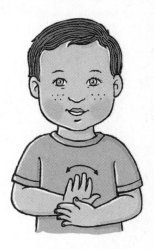

COOKIE

Use a cookie cutter on your hand.

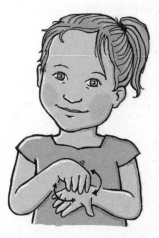

CRACKER

Tap elbow with fist.

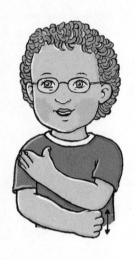

DRINK

Drink from a cup.

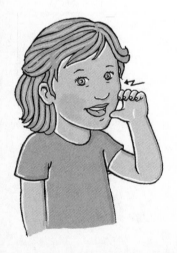

Tip: Introduce the sign for **DRINK** when you introduce your baby to a cup to help the transition to the cup. It is easier for babies to sign **DRINK** than **JUICE** or **WATER**, so consider using this sign and the generic word "drink" for anything that is not in a bottle. Learn signs for **WATER** and **JUICE** if you want to differentiate the type of drink.

JUICE

Trace the letter "J" with pinkie.

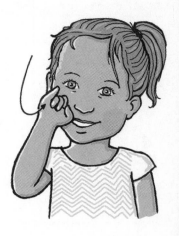

WATER

Tap three middle fingers at your lips.

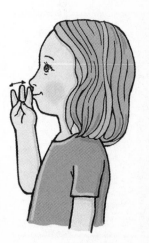

Play and Activity Signs

AIRPLANE

Fly index finger, thumb, and
pinkie through the air.

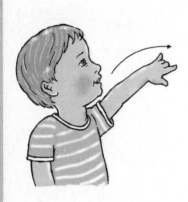

BALL

Make the shape of a ball.

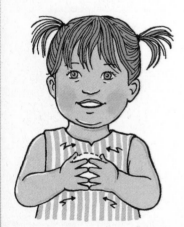

CAR

Drive a car.

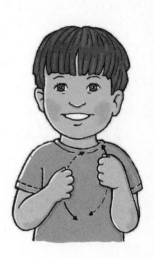

DOLL

Brush bent index finger
down nose twice.

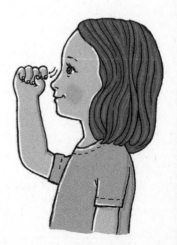

Manners Signs

HELP

Lift the fist up with the other hand, like giving a helping hand.

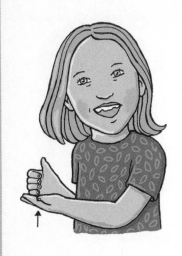

Tip: When you can see that your baby needs help doing something, ask her "Do you need some **HELP**? I will come **HELP** you." With time, she will request your help. The **HELP** sign is difficult for babies to make until they are well over a year old. Often, babies will sign **HELP** by tapping two hands on their chest.

PET (SOFT TOUCH)

Stroke the back of the hand.

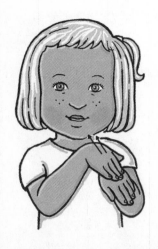

Tip: Use this sign and demonstrate how to pet an animal or stroke another child.

TOUCH

Touch the back of the hand
with your middle finger.

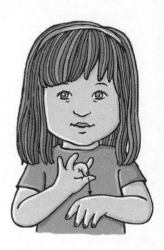

Personal Care Signs

CLEAN

Swipe one hand over the
other like cleaning.

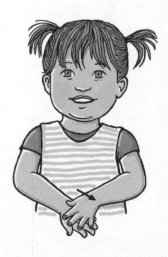

CLOTHES/GET DRESSED

Brush both hands down your chest.

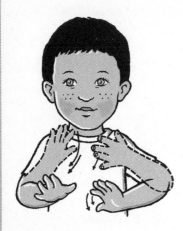

COAT

Put coat on.

PACIFIER

Place the pacifier in the mouth.

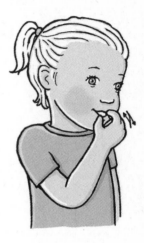

PANTS

Show each of the legs of the pants.

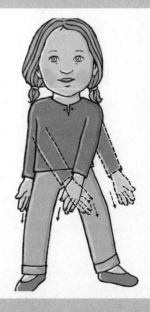

SHIRT

Pinch your shirt.

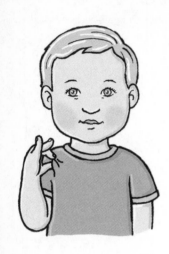

SHOES

Knock fists together.

SOCKS

Move index fingers back and
forth like knitting socks.

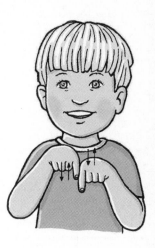

WASH HAIR

Wash your hair.

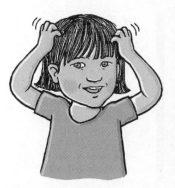

WASH/WASH HANDS

Rub hands together like washing them.

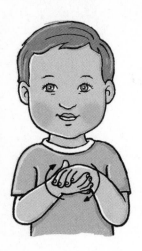

ZIPPER

Zip up your jacket.

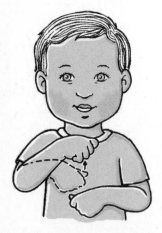

Animal Signs

ANIMAL

Put fingers on chest and
move hands like wings.

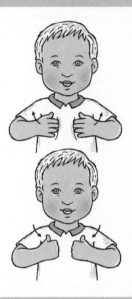

BEAR

Cross hands and scratch your chest.

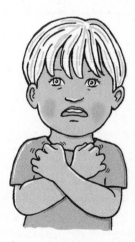

BIRD

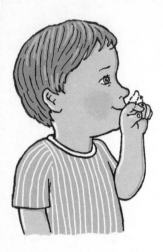

Open and close index finger
and thumb like a bird's beak.

CAT

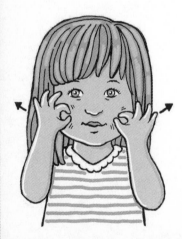

Trace the cat's whiskers on your face.

COW

Stick out pinkie like a horn
and twist the hand.

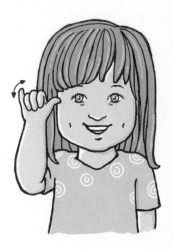

DOG

Pat your leg to call the dog.

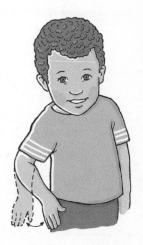

DUCK

Tap thumb with index and middle
fingers like a duck's bill.

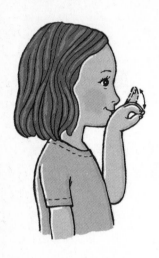

FISH

Wiggle hand like a fish swimming.

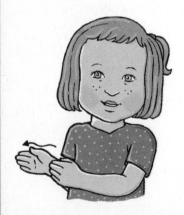

FROG

Flick fingers under chin like
frog's throat puffing.

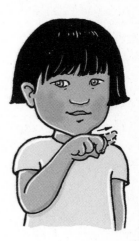

HORSE

Bend two fingers next to
forehead like a horse's ear.

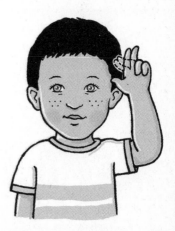

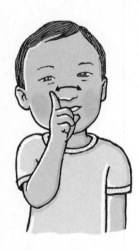

MOUSE

Rub index finger across
scrunched nose.

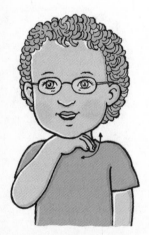

PIG

Open and close hand under chin.

RABBIT

Wiggle fingers like rabbit ears.

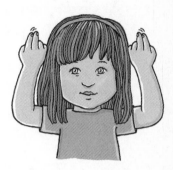

SHEEP

Use a scissors motion to "shear wool" on inside of arm.

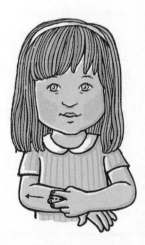

Family and Friend Signs

BABY

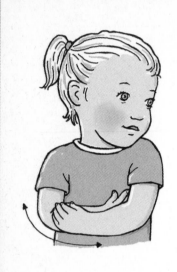

Rock a baby in your arms.

DAD

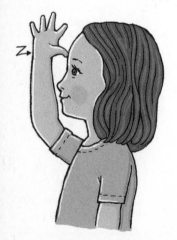

Tap thumb on your forehead.

MOM

Tap thumb on your chin.

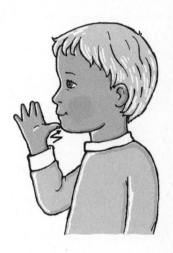

Weather/Outdoor Signs

MOON

Make a crescent moon and put it up in the sky.

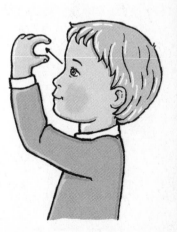

RAIN

Hands and fingers move down
like sheets of falling rain.

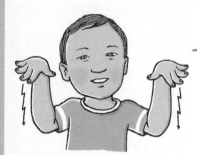

SNOW

Fingers wiggle as hands move down.

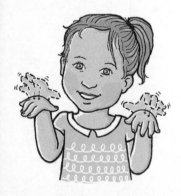

STARS

Move index fingers back and
forth like shooting stars.

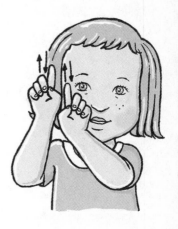

SUN

Make a circle like the sun
and then show its rays.

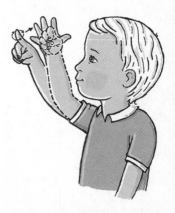

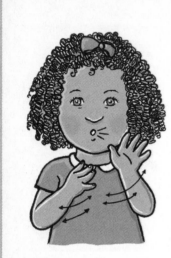

WIND

Swing hands from side to side.

ESSENTIAL SIGNS (EIGHT TO TWELVE MONTHS)

Here are the ten essential signs to learn and teach your baby at eight to twelve months:

1. APPLE (see page 51)
2. BANANA (see page 51)
3. CEREAL (see page 52)
4. DRINK (see page 54)
5. BALL (see page 56)
6. DOLL (see page 57)
7. CAT (see page 66)
8. DOG (see page 67)
9. CAR (see page 57)
10. HELP (see page 58)

CHAPTER FOUR

LET'S COMMUNICATE!—
THIRTEEN TO
EIGHTEEN MONTHS

FOR MOST BABIES, THE PERIOD from thirteen to eighteen months is a time of extensive movement and memory development. Your baby is now walking about, discovering the world around him. He has a lot to learn, and sometimes it seems like he wants to learn it all in one day.

During this time, his ability to remember things and recall information increases greatly. He now knows that you will return when you leave him for a while. He understands that when his **BEAR** is not in his sight, it is somewhere else (object permanence) and that he can go look for it. His need to express his wants and desires is also growing during this time, outpacing his verbal abilities to express himself. Signing will help him communicate and keep his frustration to a minimum.

In this chapter, we'll take a look at the following:

* How your baby is developing from thirteen to eighteen months
* How reading helps his development
* How your baby's signing abilities will explode
* How your baby's independence can be influenced by signing
* Specific activities to use during this period

Just beginning now? You can expect your baby to sign as quickly as a week or two after you begin signing. Start with signs that will motivate your child, such as food signs and other signs related to activities he enjoys. Read the previous chapters for tips and signs.

SO WHAT'S HAPPENING NOW?

Your baby is now working on the big things such as walking, jumping, and talking. You might be surprised by how much your baby will change during this period.

Motor Development

By eighteen months, you will notice that your baby's steps are smoother. She will easily navigate around obstacles instead of tripping over them. Much of the improvement in motor development occurs because her brain now has more myelin—a dense, fatty substance that helps neurons send and receive messages faster and more clearly. Myelin also helps your baby's hand coordination and manual dexterity so your baby can sign more complex signs involving two hands and slight movements.

Language Development

Your baby's language abilities are growing quickly. You can now give him simple directions such as "Give me your **BOOK**," and he can comply. *Whether* he will comply is a different matter. Babies are beginning to understand their autonomy from their parents at this age, and this feeling of independence is often expressed by refusing to comply with a parental request.

You will find that your baby knows many signs and words. The average child who does not sign will be able to understand ten to fifteen frequently used words. Babies who sign with their parents can usually sign at least this many signs and often as many as one hundred signs. This means that your baby has the ability to understand ten times more words because you sign with him than if you did not sign with him. He can now easily point to a picture in a book when you ask him "**WHERE** is the…?" and make the correct sign. He may even know how to say the word or make a sound associated with the word.

His vocabulary will grow quickly during this time, but his pronunciation can't keep pace. Fortunately he can sign and will quickly learn a lot of new signs during this time. If your baby does try to speak, resist the temptation to correct his pronunciation. Most babies mispronounce their words, and often babies will continue to sign words that they have learned to say because the pronunciation is so difficult. Just continue to speak and sign with your baby and use the correct pronunciation. This works better than correcting his pronunciation ever would. Your baby will eventually transition from signing to a signing/speech combination and finally to speech alone.

Note: Your baby may try to communicate whole thoughts through single words or signs. **BALL**, for example, may mean "Look at the ball," "I want the ball," or "Where is the ball?" You can clarify this by asking your baby questions and looking at his other signals. For example, does he sign **SLEEP** but shake his head no? He might be saying that he does not want to go to sleep. Your conversations will grow in complexity and interest for both you and your baby.

Cognitive Development

The area of your baby's brain called the hippocampus has matured enough for her to recall actions and events that occurred a few hours or even a day earlier (*deferred imitation*). You might show your baby a new sign that she does not repeat immediately. But she might display it in some form later in the day or week when you least expect it.

Your baby loves to do the same activities over and over again, and repetition is a very important learning tool. When things repeat or have a consistent pattern, your baby learns to expect or anticipate the outcome. Once your baby learns the pattern, she can concentrate on learning the details, such as the names of the animals. Embrace repetition. Your baby will probably love the same few books no matter how extensive her choices are. Use repetition to your advantage when you want to show new signs. If you have been signing just a few signs when you read her favorite book, add in a few more. Because she is already familiar with the text, adding a new sign adds a dimension of learning for her based on what she already knows.

Social Development

Your baby may have a hard time controlling his feelings and emotions at this time—this is the onset of the terrible twos, which actually start in the middle of the second year of life. This frustration stems from an inability to express needs, desires, and intensifying emotions. Signing will help your baby express his needs, wants, and feelings and should lessen the number of tantrums you experience.

Your baby is also just learning how to control his behavior (*inhibition*). Even if he knows that biting a friend is unacceptable, he may not be able to override the initial desire to bite. Inhibition is thought to be a function of the brain's frontal lobes, which are now undergoing a great deal of maturation. Additionally, if babies have no way to express themselves, their ability to control their behavior is limited. When a baby learns to sign and can express his feelings, he can begin to learn to control his behavior. Expressing how he feels and having you validate these feelings can defuse the situation and allow your baby to feel validated.

Even though you give your baby ways to express himself through signing, tantrums will come. This is a natural process of learning that helps him learn to cope with and get through difficult situations. Sympathize with your baby when he has a meltdown. Let him know that the behavior is unacceptable but that you still love him. This will give him the stability to learn to deal with his emotions and understand the rules. Make sure that the consequences of his actions are clear and appropriate for the situation.

READ TO YOUR BABY

It cannot be stressed enough that reading to your baby is paramount. Literacy will open more doors for him than you can imagine. Experts suggest fifteen to twenty minutes of reading every day has long-term benefits for your baby's learning abilities. The following is a list of suggested books that can be signed. It's okay if you read the same three to four books over and over again. Babies love repetition.

General

* *More Please* by Nancy Cadjan (the first book written specifically for children to sign from beginning to end)
* *Goodnight Moon* by Margaret Wise Brown
* *Peek-a WHO?* By Nina Laden
* *Show Me!* by Tom Tracy
* *My First Body Board Book* by DK Publishing
* *My First Word Book* by DK Publishing
* *Pat the Bunny* by Dorothy Kunhardt
* *Let's Play* by Leo Lionni

Food

* *The Very Hungry Caterpillar* by Eric Carle
* *Lunch* by Denise Fleming
* *Today Is Monday* by Eric Carle

Animals

* *Moo, Baa, La La La!* by Sandra Boynton
* *Brown Bear, Brown Bear* by Eric Carle
* *Good Night, Gorilla* by Peggy Rathmann
* *Barnyard Dance!* by Sandra Boynton
* *Does a Kangaroo Have a Mother?* by Eric Carle
* *There Was an Old Lady Who Swallowed a Fly* by Simms Taback

Routine

* *Hey! Wake Up!* by Sandra Boynton
* *The Going to Bed Book* by Sandra Boynton
* *Pajama Time* by Sandra Boynton
* *10 Minutes till Bedtime* by Peggy Rathmann
* *Clifford's Bedtime* by Norman Bridwell

Emotions/Behavior

* *Curious George's Are You Curious?* by H. A. Rey
* *Hands Are Not for Hitting* by Martine Agassi
* *I Love Hugs* by Lara Jones
* *Excuse Me!* by Karen Katz
* *Hug* by Jez Alborough
* *Kiss Kiss!* by Margaret Wild
* *Today I Feel Silly and Other Moods That Make My Day* by Jamie Lee Curtis

Colors/Descriptors

* *Blue Hat, Green Hat* by Sandra Boynton
* *Oh My Oh My Oh Dinosaurs!* by Sandra Boynton
* *What Makes a Rainbow?* by Betty Ann Schwartz

THE SIGNING EXPLOSION

> ### TIPS FOR SIGNING SUCCESS
>
> * Sign anything you know in the story and ask your baby to sign what he knows.
> * Ask your baby questions about what is happening in the book.
> * Choose books your baby can sign.
> * Choose picture-only books and tell your own story.
> * If the text is too hard for your baby, just use the pictures to tell your own story.
> * Read books that have to do with activities you do often.

Your baby now has the manual dexterity and cognitive abilities she needs to express what she needs with signs. She may also be speaking a few words, but it could be several months before she can communicate equally as well in speech as she can with signing. This is the time when most babies begin to explode with signs: they increase the number of signs they make and the contexts they use them in. They may also begin to use two-sign combinations, such as **MORE MILK**.

You can help your baby learn signs with a few of these strategies:

* Add sounds to your signs and words. When you sign **ELEPHANT**, make a trumpeting sound. This helps your baby focus.
* Sign near or on the object you are signing about. Make the sign for **BEAR** right on the bear. Your baby sees the sign and the object it represents together. You can even add a bear growl.
* Sign the signs right on your baby. Say "Do you love your **BEAR**?" Sign **BEAR** right on your baby's chest.

✳ Ask your baby to make a choice. When you ask her whether she wants an **APPLE** or a **BANANA** to eat, she needs to communicate with you. She may choose to point or sign the fruit she wants. Either way, she is learning that communication gets her what she wants.

> One issue that arises during the signing explosion is that a lot of the signs your baby makes may look the same. This is because your baby's fine motor skills may not be advanced enough to make the fine distinctions between movements. You will generally be able to tell what the sign is in context.

Look for Signing Opportunities

Timing is everything. If your baby is interested, happy, or calm, he will be more receptive to seeing and learning a sign than when he is tired or interested in something else. Look for the following clues for when your baby is ready to receive a sign:

✳ **Stares at an object with interest:** Introduce the sign for the object. If he sees a dog, say "You see the **DOG**? Yes, that is a **DOG**."

✳ **Moves toward an object:** His movement is an outward expression of his interest. If he goes for a doll, say "Do you like that **DOLL**?"

✳ **Becomes intent or very excited about something:** Introduce signs to help him understand what he is excited about. Your baby sees his first monkey at the zoo. Say "That's a **MONKEY** swinging on the branch."

✳ **Starts getting frustrated because he can't express himself or get what he needs:** Sometimes the moment between the calm and the frustration is a perfect time to introduce a sign. If you are eating cheese and you can tell he wants to try it, ask him "Do you want to try the **CHEESE**?"

Converse with Your Baby

Your goal is to use sign language to help bridge the time before she can speak so that you can start to communicate now. For parents, talking to their baby is sometimes difficult because they don't know how to talk to someone who can't really talk back.

Here are three ways you can have a conversation even when she can't talk back.

* *Parallel talk* is talking about what you see. Describe what your baby is doing. She can hear the words that go with the activities she is participating in: "You are **PLAYING** with the **DOLL**. Does your **BABY** want some **MILK**?"
* *Self talk* is talking about what you are doing. Your baby watches you and what you are doing: "I am **WASHING** my hands. Now I am **COOKING** dinner." When you narrate what you are doing, you give her words and signs for the things she sees you do.
* *Stretch talk* or *expansion* is adding to what your baby is saying or signing. If she signs **EAT**, you say "You want to **EAT**? How about some **APPLES**? Let me put some **APPLES** on your plate." You have stretched her request for food and added a specific type of food—apples—and a place to put the food—a plate.

She will use the words she learns through parallel talk, self talk, and stretch talk later when she is ready to talk about similar things. Her first sentences in sign and speech will be *telegraphic*, meaning that they will leave out words such as "a" and "the." **MORE DRINK** is a common example.

DEALING WITH YOUR BABY'S INDEPENDENCE

Your baby now sees things he wants to do, places he wants to go, or things he wants to get. If he cannot tell you what his plans are, generally, everything ends in a tantrum. If you are lucky enough to guess, you might avoid one. If you see your baby heading to do something, ask him to tell you what he wants and see if he can explain himself using signs. Shelly, mother of fourteen-month-old Henry, explains, "We were at the park, and I noticed that Henry was walking away from everyone. I wondered why. I asked him, and he turned around and looked at me and signed **SLIDE**. When I looked in the direction he was headed, there was a big blue slide just like one we had. He was heading toward the slide to have fun just like we do at home. Pretty amazing that a fourteen-month-old can tell you he wants to go for a slide." Without signing, Shelly might have guessed why Henry was taking off away from his friends and family, but with signing, she knew exactly where Henry was going and why. She had a window into his interests.

Important: Don't give your child an option if you really need him to do something. This applies in all situations. If you need him to do something or you must do something, make a statement: "We are going to the store." Don't say "Do you want to go to the store?" If you ask a question, you are implying choice. If there is no choice, don't ask it as a question.

Encourage Signing, Not Screaming

Your baby now understands that there are specific things she wants and likes or does not. For parents who do not sign with their babies, this may mean a lot of screaming and head scratching—screaming on the baby's part and head scratching on the parent's part. When you show your baby the signs for the things she wants, you have a way to bypass the frustration.

As your baby's need to express herself increases in parallel with her growing independence and desire to learn about her world, there will be many instances where she needs to communicate something to you. You have taught your baby to sign to help her explain her needs, but she will not always remember that she has the skill, and she may start to cry. Whenever you sense that she wants something but can't get her point across, ask her to "Tell me with your hands." This might help her remember that she knows how to communicate with you in a more effective manner than screaming.

You can also use "Tell me with your hands" for times when your child tries to use spoken words but they are not clear. Tricia read to her son Dallin every day before nap time. "When he was eighteen months old, he was starting to replace signs with words and was trying to tell me something that he wanted. I did not understand. He looked up at me disgusted and signed **BOOK**." He was ready for his book and his nap. Without the sign, Dallin probably would have broken into tears. By helping your baby to realize that he has a way to clarify his point and ensure that he is getting it across, you can skip many of the tantrums caused when children feel they are powerless to get what they need.

Teach Good Manners

Start to show your baby the signs that will help him have good manners and play well with other children by using these signs yourself when you speak with him. This is called *modeling*. Babies learn by example, so when you speak with your baby, say such things as "**PLEASE** may I **PLAY** with your **DOLL**?" or "**THANK YOU** for helping me **CHANGE** your diaper."

It may sound strange to talk this way, but it does two things. It introduces your baby to the language of good manners, and it gives him a chance to feel the effects of them. When you treat your baby with respect and ask him if you can play with his doll and thank him for his cooperation when changing diapers, you respect his individuality. He will internalize this type of interaction and learn to treat others the same way. Additionally, because you are showing your baby the signs for things such as **PLEASE** and **THANK YOU**, he has a way to conceptualize these abstract ideas and use them in his life. Other signs that help introduce the concept of good manners are **HELP**, **STOP**,

NO TOUCH, **SOFT TOUCH**, and **SHARE**. If your baby is doing something that you want him to stop doing, use the sign **STOP** instead of **NO**.

Some children may be able to sign fifty to one hundred signs while others only know one or two signs. The consistency with which you sign with your baby makes a lot of difference, but your baby also has his own personal rhythms and reasons for signing. Some children see signing as a tool only to use to get what they need, and others enjoy the process of signing. Your baby could be more interested in conquering some physical milestone at the moment, or he might just be more contemplative before he signs.

Babies do not yet understand the multiple meanings of the word **NO** ("No, do not do that" versus "No, I don't have one of those"). **STOP** is a more direct way to explain that you want the behavior to stop.

SIGN MORE AND SIGN OFTEN

The sky is the limit when it comes to signing now. You can introduce signs for anything your baby is interested in—and she will be interested in everything. Take your baby's interests and run with them. Sign what you know and learn as you go.

* Place a piece of dry cereal on her high chair. When she eats it, ask her "Do you want some **MORE**?" Wait until she signs **MORE** to give her another piece. Babies love to play this game and love to be "in charge."

* Hide an object such as a book partially behind your back so your baby can still see it. Then say "**WHERE** is the **BOOK**? I can't find it. **WHERE** did it go?"

* Reinforce **STOP** and **MORE** by stopping an activity and asking her whether she wants more. If you are tickling her, say "**STOP**" and then wait a few seconds and then ask whether she wants **MORE**.

* When you are finished playing and do not want to continue the

game, say "We are **ALL DONE**." This way she knows it is the end of the game.

❋ When you sign and say the name of the animal, add the sound that animal makes. These sounds also allow your baby to practice the basics of speech and help her develop the muscles she needs to speak.

❋ Visit a pet store and use the signs for **FROG**, **RABBIT**, **CAT**, **DOG**, **FISH**, and **BIRD**.

❋ Take a walk around the neighborhood with your baby and show her **HOUSE**, **TREE**, and **FLOWER**. You could even look at the **INSECTS** and listen to the **BIRDS**. If a **CAR** goes by or you hear an **AIRPLANE** or a **HELICOPTER**, let her know what these things are by naming and signing them.

❋ Use clear containers to "hide" a toy and then ask "**WHERE** is the **BALL**? Can you find the **BALL**?" Say "Let's look in here." Then, when your baby has found the ball, congratulate her. "You found the **BALL**! **THANK YOU**!" As your hide-and-seek game becomes more sophisticated, you can add other signs to your sentences such as **PLEASE** and **HELP**.

❋ Take one of her stuffed animals (not her favorite one if you think she may cry when it gets "hurt") and have it accidentally fall down. Say "Oh, that must have **HURT**." Alternatively, you can ask the stuffed animal "**WHERE** does it **HURT**?" Then pretend you are the stuffed animal and speak in a high voice and say "It **HURTS** here" and sign where on the animal it hurts. If that place requires a Band-Aid, have your baby put one on. You can extend the game to include stomachaches and teething pain.

❋ If you struggle with brushing teeth, brush the teeth of your baby's dolls and bears. Say "See how the bear **BRUSHES** his **TEETH**? **BRUSH** them up and down. Now they are so clean."

✳ A fun ritual to help your baby understand that it's time for bed is to have a **SLEEP** walk in which you say good night to your baby's favorite things around the house. When you get to each thing, say **SLEEP BEAR, SLEEP BALL, SLEEP** train, etc. By the time you get to your baby's bed, she should be ready to sleep. You can also put her favorite stuffed animals to **BED**. By putting her bears to **BED**, she sees that everyone is going to bed and prepares herself for sleep.

As you approach eighteen months, you may want to look ahead to the signs in the next chapter. There are many signs for emotions and actions that will come in handy when your baby is ready for them. Or if you need a specific sign, check out the list of signs on page 197.

ALL YOU NEED (THIRTEEN TO EIGHTEEN MONTHS)

○ Sign when you read and let your baby sign what he knows while reading.

○ Ask your baby questions while reading so he can sign back or point out things in the book.

○ Combine signs together and add descriptors.

○ Add sounds to your signs and words.

○ Sign near or on the object you are signing about.

○ Sign the signs right on your baby.

○ Ask your baby to make a choice.

○ Show him a sign when he stares at an object with interest, moves toward an object, or becomes intent or very excited about something.

○ The moment before frustration when your baby wants something is a perfect time to introduce a sign.

○ Use parallel talk, self talk, and stretch talk to keep the conversation going.

○ Encourage good manners with signs.

SIGNS FOR THIRTEEN TO EIGHTEEN MONTHS
Food Signs

BEANS

Twist the bean open.

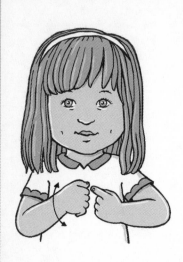

BERRY

Twist the berry off your pinkie.

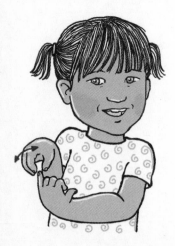

CARROT

Bite a carrot.

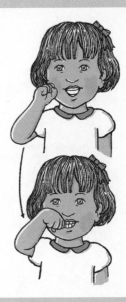

CHICKEN

Show the beak and then peck at the ground.

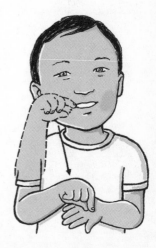

CORN

Eat a cob of corn.

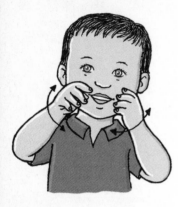

EGG

Tap fingers together like breaking and opening an egg.

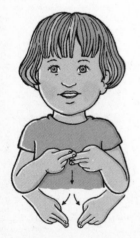

FRUIT

Twist thumb and index finger
at the side of the mouth.

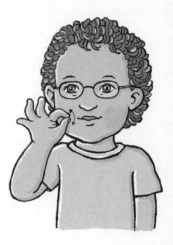

GRAPES

Tap bent hands down other hand to
show the clusters on the grapevine.

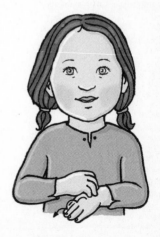

MEAT

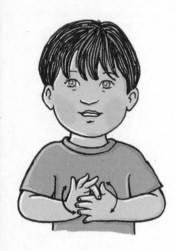

Pinch skin between thumb and index finger and wiggle pinching hand.

ORANGE

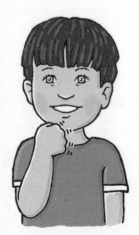

Squeeze orange near mouth.

PEACH

Feel the peach fuzz on your cheek.

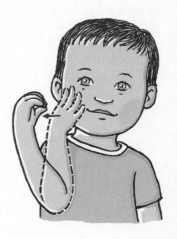

PEAR

Show the shape of a
pear on your hand.

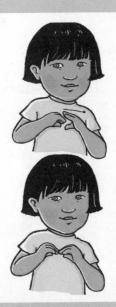

PEAS

Show the peas in the pod.

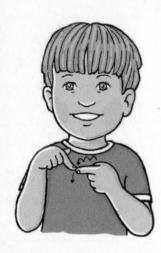

POTATO

Stick a fork in the potato.

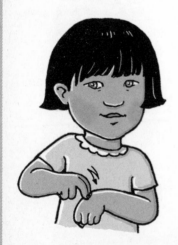

RICE

Scoop rice out of hand with crossed fingers.

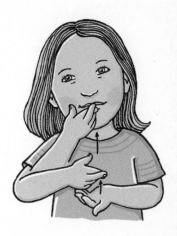

SPAGHETTI

Circle pinkies as they move away from each other.

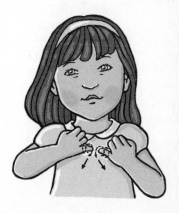

SPOON

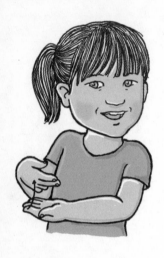

Scoop with two fingers
like picking up food.

VEGETABLE

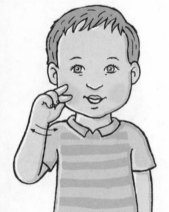

Twist index and middle fingers
at the side of the mouth.

Action Signs

CATCH

Catch something in the air.

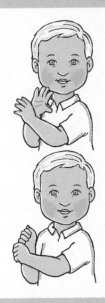

CRY

Show the falling tears with fingers.

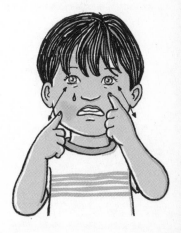

FALL DOWN

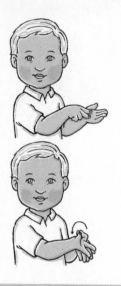

Stand index and middle fingers on
the hand and then "fall down."

GO

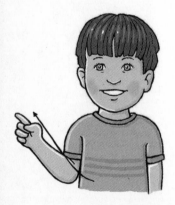

Point index finger the way
you want to go.

HEAR/LISTEN

Put hand to ear like you are
listening to something.

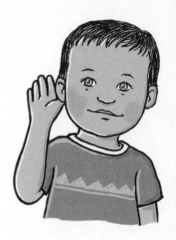

HIDE

Take the secret from your lips and
hide it under the other hand.

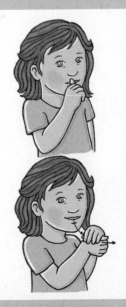

JUMP

Bounce fingers on the
palm of the hand.

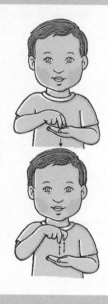

SWING

Fold fingers over like legs sitting on
a chair, then swing back and forth.

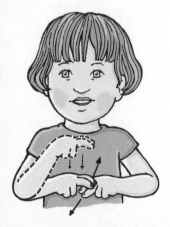

THROW

Throw something.

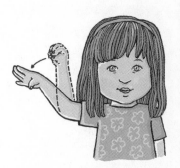

TICKLE

Tickle.

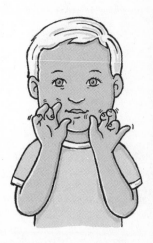

WALK

Shuffle hands like walking.

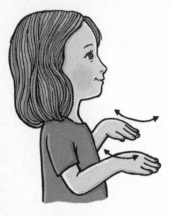

Manners Signs

HURT

Touch index fingers together
at the location of the pain.

Tip: **HURT** is a handy sign because you sign it wherever something hurts. If you have a headache, you sign **HURT** at your head. If you have fallen and hurt your leg, you sign **HURT** at the point where the scrape is. Also, it helps when you have to go to the doctor for shots or other procedures.

SHARE

Pass one hand over vertical fingers of other hand like dividing something.

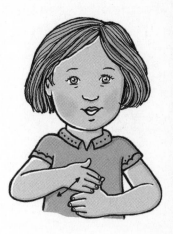

STOP

Create a barrier on your hand.

Tip: Use the sign **STOP** instead of saying no, which babies often ignore. If he is reaching for something that is off limits, say and sign **STOP** to help him know that it is off limits.

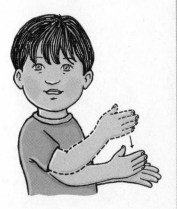

Personal Care Signs

BRUSH TEETH

Brush your teeth.

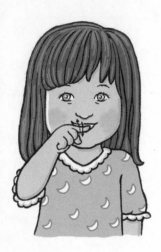

POTTY

Tuck your thumb under your index finger and then shake it.

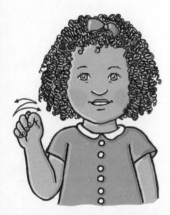

Household Signs

BALLOON

Show the balloon growing
bigger as you blow it up.

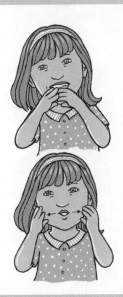

BUBBLES

Wiggle fingers while moving
hands from waist to neck.

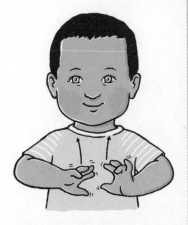

DINOSAUR

Point index finger and bounce
it up the other arm.

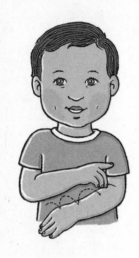

FLOWER

Smell the flower at your nose.

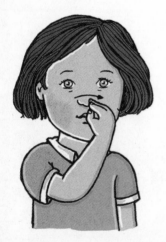

HELICOPTER

Rest hand on top of index finger,
then rock hand side to side.

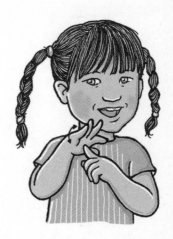

OUT/OUTSIDE

Take something out of a container.

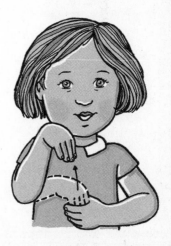

TELEPHONE

Make a phone with your thumb
and pinkie at the ear.

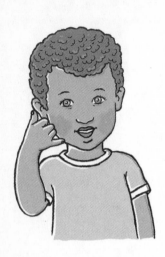

TOYS

Tuck thumbs under index
fingers and twist hands.

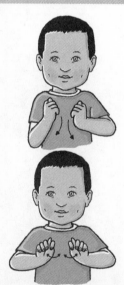

TREE

Form a tree with your arm and hand, then twist hand like swaying in the wind.

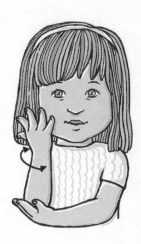

Bedtime Signs

BLANKET

Move hands like pulling a blanket up to your chest.

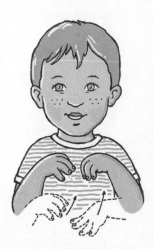

BRUSH HAIR

Brush your hair.

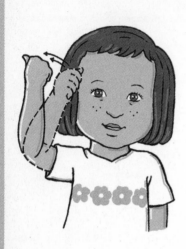

DREAM

Wiggle index finger out from head.

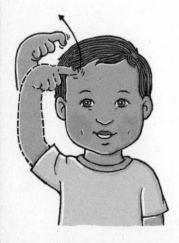

PAJAMAS

Use two signs: **SLEEP** and **CLOTHES**.

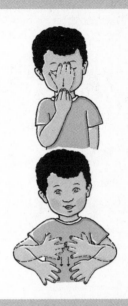

PILLOW

Fluff the pillow at the side of your head.

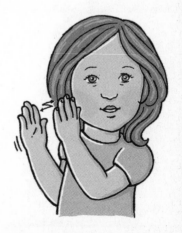

Animal Signs

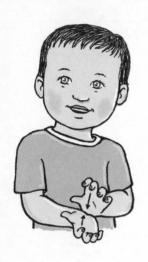

ALLIGATOR

Open and close two hands together like alligator's mouth.

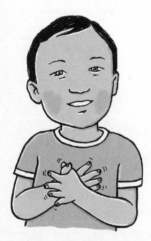

BUTTERFLY

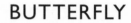

Hook thumbs together and flap hands like wings.

ELEPHANT

Move curved hand from nose
down to show elephant's trunk.

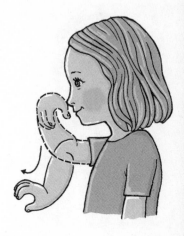

GIRAFFE

Show the giraffe's long neck.

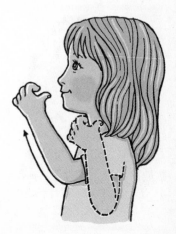

INSECT

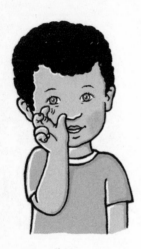

Wiggle two fingers in front of
nose like an insect's antenna.

KANGAROO

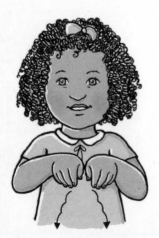

Make both hands hop like a kangaroo.

LION

Move hand back over the head
to show the lion's mane.

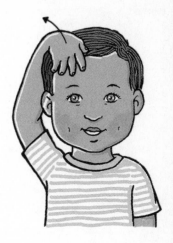

MONKEY

Scratch under your arms
like a monkey.

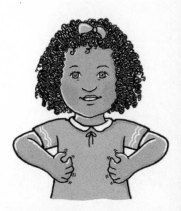

SPIDER

Cross hands, interlock pinkies,
and wiggle fingers.

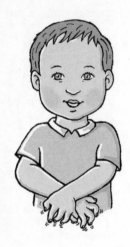

SQUIRREL

Tap two fingers like squirrel's
teeth opening and closing.

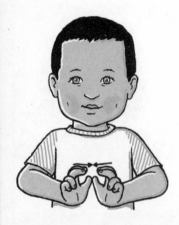

TIGER

Move fingers across face to
show the tiger's stripes.

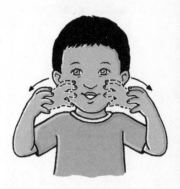

TURTLE

Curve top hand like a shell and
wiggle thumb like a turtle's head.

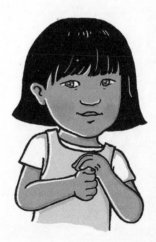

Family and Friend Signs

BOY

Pinch the bill of a baseball cap.

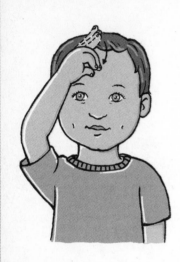

BROTHER

Touch thumb at forehead, then bring down to cross the wrist on the other hand.

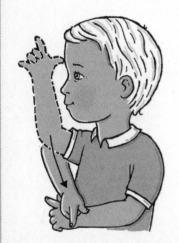

FAMILY

Touch thumb and index fingers together,
then move to make a family circle.

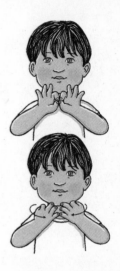

FRIEND

Hook index fingers together
and then switch them.

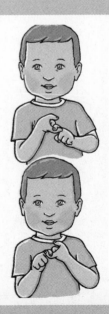

GIRL

Trace the girl's bonnet strings with thumb.

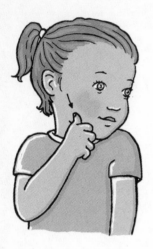

GRANDFATHER

Touch thumb to forehead, then bounce hand forward twice.

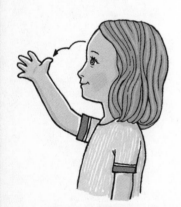

GRANDMOTHER

Touch thumb to chin, then
bounce hand forward twice.

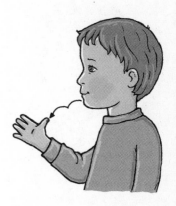

SISTER

Touch thumb at chin, then bring down
to cross the wrist on the other hand.

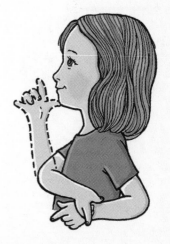

Descriptor Signs

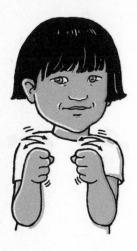

COLD

Make two fists and shake
them like you're shivering.

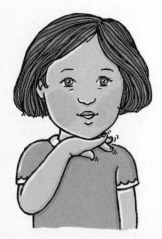

DIRTY

Wiggle fingers under chin.

HOT

Take something hot out of mouth.

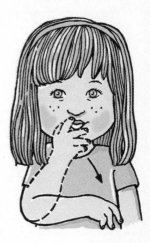

ESSENTIAL SIGNS (THIRTEEN TO EIGHTEEN MONTHS)

Here are the fifteen essential signs to learn and teach your baby at thirteen to eighteen months:

1.   SHARE (see page 109)
2.   STOP (see page 109)
3.   HURT (see page 108)
4.   WALK (see page 108)
5.   JUMP (see page 106)
6.   BRUSH TEETH (see page 110)
7.   WASH HANDS (see page 64)
8.   POTTY (see page 110)
9.   TELEPHONE (see page 114)
10. FLOWER (see page 112)
11. TREE (see page 115)
12. FRUIT (see page 97)
13. CHICKEN (see page 95)
14. VEGETABLE (see page 102)
15. INSECT (see page 120)

CHAPTER FIVE

I CAN TALK AND SIGN!— NINETEEN TO TWENTY- FOUR MONTHS

IF YOUR CHILD HAS NOT started to talk yet, she will probably do so now. But this is *not* the time to stop signing, because it will be several months until your child can express herself easily. You will spend the next several months transitioning from signing and speaking to just speaking. In fact, don't be surprised if your child is still signing at two and a half—many are as they continue to learn.

In this chapter, we'll take a look at the following:

* How your child is developing from nineteen to twenty-four months
* How to incorporate signing and speaking at the same time
* How to expand language learning
* How to continue teaching good manners and develop emotional maturity
* Specific activities to use during this period

Just beginning now? If you are just beginning to sign with your child, great! You can expect your child to sign back as quickly as a few days or a week after you begin signing. Start with signs that will motivate your child, such as food and other signs related to activities he enjoys.

SO WHAT'S HAPPENING NOW?

At this age, your child is becoming very coordinated and is learning to speak in simple sentences and express her emotions. This is still the time of the terrible twos, but signing will lessen the impact on you and your child.

Motor Development

Your child is working on the fine motor skills that involve the small muscles in her fingers, hands, and wrists, such as drawing, fitting shapes in a shape sorter, and using a spoon and fork. Her cerebellum, an area of the brain that is important for the timing and coordination of most motor tasks, is also developing and further aids your child's abilities. If your child is not interested in sitting and drawing or writing, don't worry. All forms of fine motor activity—including signing—provide stimulation for her developing brain and motor system.

Movement is necessary and extremely important to her sense of well-being. If you confine her too much, she is likely to throw a tantrum. She needs the freedom to move so that she can improve her gross motor skills, the use of the large muscles of the body. When it is safe and appropriate, let her explore her surroundings. It will help her refine her coordination, gain confidence in moving her body through space, release some of her energy, and develop new motor skills such as running, jumping, and climbing. Each new motor skill contributes to your child's sense of mastery and her growing feeling of competence.

Language Development

The number of words a child uses between nineteen and twenty-four months is related to several factors, such as gender, personality (whether he is outgoing or shy), family size, and so forth. As we've already seen, babies who sign with their parents generally speak sooner and have larger vocabularies than their counterparts who do not sign. The average child who does not sign says around fifty words at age two, while babies who sign often speak and/or sign between one hundred fifty and three hundred words by this age.

The speed at which his vocabulary grows increases exponentially once your child feels comfortable and has a large enough vocabulary to have his basic needs met (somewhere between thirty and sixty words in sign and speech). This can occur as early as fourteen months in babies who sign. Once he reaches this critical mass, he begins adding new words or signs to his vocabulary every day. If your child has not already started to, he will put together two- and three-word sentences, both in sign and words. Often, babies who sign have been creating two- and three-word sentences in sign and speech for months, but if not, look for this milestone.

The amount of language used in conversation with children influences their rate of verbal language development. The more words a child hears while engaged in conversations, the larger his vocabulary will be and the faster it will continue to grow. This is one reason why babies who sign speak sooner and have larger vocabularies than babies who do not—their parents engage them in conversations at an earlier age and more often. Sara was amazed one day when her eighteen-month-old son commented on the weather. "We stepped out of the grocery store, and he looked into the sky and said, 'Hey Dad, it's a cloudy day.' My jaw dropped; I couldn't believe that he said a full, understandable sentence and even used the correct verb tense."

Make sure you take time to listen to your child. Put the phone down and turn off the computer. If his speech is unclear, try to understand him and use sign to help him express himself. Don't assume you know what he is saying, and don't speak for him. By giving him the chance to speak, you give him important practice. You can clarify things by restating what he says and asking him whether you got the correct message.

Cognitive Development

At this age, your child learns primarily through hands-on experiences, and her cognitive development is directly related to how many experiences she has. Telling your child about things is not as powerful as allowing her to experience them herself. Giving her a wide variety of sensory, motor, and pretend play opportunities is a great way to support her development and doesn't require that you teach her directly. Let her mix paint colors to see that yellow and blue make green.

Your child now understands that symbols can stand for objects and experiences, a concept called *symbolic representation*. She will begin to extend this understanding to symbolic thought and pretend play. She will talk into a toy phone with someone she imagines is on the line or make dinner out of blocks. Symbolic thought is an important step in learning to read and write, and she will soon be able to understand that letters and words represent thoughts.

Some children who sign learn the alphabet at this age without a parent's help. This higher cognitive function is a direct result of your child's ability to understand symbolic representation and use symbolic thought related to the symbolic nature of signing. When my son was about sixteen months old, he had a bad cold, and we spent the entire day in bed. To break up the day, we watched a *Sesame Street* video about the alphabet a few times. When he got up that evening, he walked to the refrigerator and noticed that there were three letters on it. He matter-of-factly said, "C, R, Z." I was shocked, because I had never tried teaching him the alphabet. Within the next few weeks, he learned the entire alphabet on his own and began reading letters from signs on buildings when we went shopping.

Social Development

Your child is now developing an awareness of self. He knows that there is not only a "me" but also a "mine." Your child may become very possessive of his toys and even of his parents. This can lead to conflicts, as this is also a time when babies begin to socialize and play in groups. Keep in mind your child's possessiveness is a way for him to express his independence and autonomy. Understanding this makes understanding his behavior easier. He is not trying to be a brat; he is simply working out his understanding of self.

Avert problems by explaining "This is your doll, but can we **SHARE** it with Ella for two minutes?" When he knows that you know that the doll is his, he may be more willing to share it. Self-control is still developing at this age. He understands you when you tell him not to take from others, but his lack of self-control may cause him to take it anyway. Self-control comes with time and brain maturation. It is perfectly okay if he has some special toys he does not share with others. Don't take these to a playdate, and hide them when friends visit.

When your child has a greater sense that he can make things happen, he has a greater sense of self-competence. You can enhance this sense of self-competence and self-esteem by giving your child simple choices between two equal things, such as two different shirts or two types of fruit. He wants to have a say in his life. When he feels that he has some control, he is less likely to have temper tantrums.

HOW TO SIGN AND SPEAK AT THE SAME TIME

During your child's transition to spoken language, she many continue to sign words that she is able to speak. If she notices that you don't understand her, she will use a sign for clarification. Or she might use a sign as a way to underscore the importance of the word. Many mothers report that long after their children can speak clearly—even sometimes as late as four or five years old—their children will sign and say **PLEASE** whenever they really want something. Signing seems to function like an exclamation point for these children, giving them a way to add emphasis.

Like adults do sometimes, your child can lose the ability to communicate when she gets frustrated. The motor control needed to make signs requires less from your child than the motor control needed to form words. In times like these, remind your child to "use your hands" so that she remembers she can speak with signs until her ability to talk returns. Children who do not have sign language to fall back on often resort to screaming or hitting to get their point across. You will see less of this behavior if your child has a backup language system. Many preschools have begun teaching signs to children so that they will have a way to communicate when they are frustrated.

Don't worry; your child will not be hampered in her transition to spoken language by signing. The bridge you have given her remains there for her to use whenever she needs it.

EXPAND YOUR CHILD'S LANGUAGE LEARNING

Continue to expand your child's language experience through *stretch talk* (adding to what your child says). When your child initiates a conversation by signing something to you that you did not ask him about, make sure that you extend the conversation by asking him more questions or providing him with more information.

If your child comments on the fact that **DADDY** is **EATING**, you can extend the comment to a conversation by asking questions such as "**WHAT** is **DADDY EATING**?" Give your child time to answer back. If he doesn't answer back, try asking him such silly questions as "Is he **EATING BEARS** or **SHOES**?" Often silly questions prompt a response. When he tells you what Daddy is eating, confirm it for him with signs and speech. "Yes, **DADDY** is **EATING APPLES**."

Extend the language learning to a game. When you play hide-and-seek, add a linguistic element your game. Think out loud about where you might be hiding to introduce or reinforce vocabulary. Say "**WHERE** is Alexa?" and then add "Maybe she is in the pantry next to the **CRACKERS?**" The nonsense in this sentence is funny to your child, but helps her learn more complex words. She knows that there is a place where the crackers go but might not know that it is called the pantry. She is listening to you because she wants to be found, so you have a captive audience. Or play a simplified version of Simon Says. Say "Show me your nose. Show me your toes."

Finally, children at this age are beginning to enjoy language for language's sake. They begin to understand the words to rhymes and enjoy the sound of the rhymes. Now that your child knows the rhymes to the songs you sing often, change the words and signs a bit and see what she does. You can also introduce her to nonsensical books. She will begin to understand the irony in these books. Or make up funny names for things your child knows the name for. Playing with language helps children understand the rhythm of language.

CONTINUE TO DEVELOP GOOD MANNERS

You can continue to model basic good manners by signing and saying **PLEASE**, **THANK YOU**, **SORRY**, and **SHARE**. The best way to teach manners is to lead by example. Use good manners and polite language: "**DADDY, PLEASE** pass me the carrots. **THANK YOU**." If you exaggerate the **PLEASE** and **THANK YOU**, it makes the words more interesting to your child, and they are more likely to process them and use them. You can even extend the good manners lesson to play time. Have a tea party with your child's dolls or stuffed animals and use the words for good manners. Allow your child to interact and ask her dolls to **PLEASE** pass the **COOKIES**.

Praise your child when she uses any of the signs or words for good manners. She will be encouraged to continue using her good manners if she is rewarded emotionally each time. This is the age when you will start arranging playdates with other moms. If their children are also signing, look to see whether the children sign together. Often, when your child needs to ask for something, she will sign **PLEASE** to her playmates, even if she won't sign **PLEASE** with you.

Make sure that in addition to using the words and the signs, your voice and face match the word and the feeling you are trying to convey. For example, if you say **SORRY** to your child, make sure your face looks sorry and your voice sounds sorry. Exaggeration helps. If you have done something that requires an apology, make sure your child sees you sign **SORRY**. You can also teach your child to use this sign when she has done something that needs an apology.

DEVELOP EMOTIONAL MATURITY

From the day your child was born, you have probably dreaded the day when he would throw tantrums. Because you sign with him, you might have found that you have not experienced as many tantrums as parents who have children of the same age. Most tantrums occur because a child feels little sense of control, cannot get his point across, or cannot get his needs met. Signing has helped your child in this area, because he has a sense of control over his environment, he has an ability to get his point across, and he can get his needs met.

You will also notice that your child's range of emotions is growing. He is now showing you signs of pride, frustration, timidity, and also exhilaration and fierce independence. As he learns the gamut of emotions, you will need to deal with them. Sometimes, this leads to conflict and issues. Always remember *not* to mistake your child's verbal and signing abilities for emotional maturity. He might be able to talk or sign to you words that are well beyond his age, but he is still very young and emotionally immature. Allow him to be a child, and give him a chance to learn about his new emotions. If you can, avoid situations that cause problems. For example, if you know he gets edgy when he is hungry, carry snacks. Or if he is exhausted in the grocery store and heading for a meltdown, leave the cart with the manager and take him home and put him to bed. Sometimes, you have to step in and be the parent and help him before he has a meltdown. This may mean sacrificing your own schedule for his benefit.

EXPAND THE SIGNING SITUATIONS

You and your child have been signing for quite a while now, and you have an amazing repertoire of signs under your belt. You may not need to add more signs to communicate. Instead, expand the situations in which you use signs to give your child more language experiences.

* **Name That Feeling:** As your child matures into her emotions, giving each of her different feelings a name is extremely useful to help her express them. The best way to help your child identify emotions is by modeling and labeling them with words and signs. If you two are playing and laughing and being silly, you can take that opportunity to say "I feel **SILLY** and I feel **HAPPY**." That way, your child learns the words for how she is feeling too.

    You can also use books and songs to teach your child what emotions are. One book that helps teach moods and emotions is *Today I Feel Silly and Other Moods That Make My Day* by Jamie Lee Curtis. Another is *Curious George's Are You Curious?* by H. A. Rey. Or you can play the "Feeling Game." First you model what feelings look like, and then you say "Show me what **SAD** looks like. Show me what you look like when you're **HAPPY**."

* **Around Town:** Turn your experiences around town into learning experiences. A trip to the grocery store can introduce concepts and words to your child. Tell your child about what you are seeing and ask her for help. Have her tell you what the foods are, and ask her to watch

out for certain items. Say "**WHERE** are the **APPLES**?" Have her help you put the apples in the bag. Ask her "Do we need **MORE APPLES**?"

Remember to look back at the signs from previous chapters to find things you can be signing. There is also a list of all signs on page 197 so you can quickly find the sign you need.

Have her hold things that are safe for her to hold. Remember that for a trip to be successful, you should only go when your child is rested and spend only a short time. As adults, we want to get everything done at once, but children can't take that much mental stimulation and need their naps. Don't sacrifice your child's well-being to get that last errand in.

ALL YOU NEED (NINETEEN TO TWENTY-FOUR MONTHS)

- The more you talk and sign to you child, the larger her vocabulary will be.
- Your child will talk and sign during this time.
- When you child gets frustrated, remind her to use her signs.
- Help your child label her emotions with signs.
- Use your daily activities as learning experiences.

SIGNS FOR NINETEEN TO TWENTY-FOUR MONTHS
Food Signs

CAKE

Make the cake rise on hand.

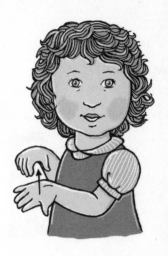

CANDY

Twist finger at cheek.

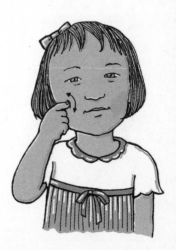

FRENCH FRIES

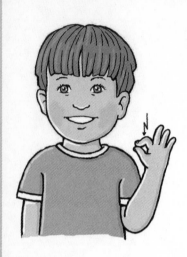

Bounce index finger and
thumb in the air.

HAMBURGER

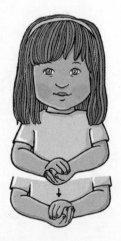

Shape a hamburger patty in your hand.

HOT DOG

Place the hot dog in the bun.

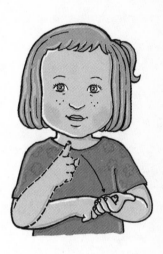

ICE CREAM

Move ice cream cone in front of mouth to lick it.

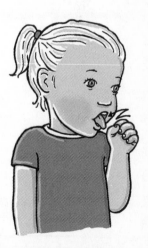

KETCHUP

Tap on the bottom of the bottle.

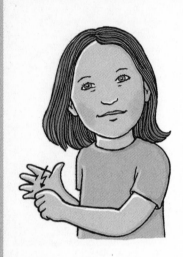

PEANUT BUTTER AND JELLY

Brush thumb against teeth, butter bread with two fingers, and then spread jelly with pinkie.

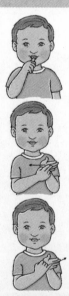

PIE

Cut the pie into slices on your hand.

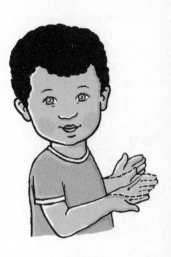

PIZZA

Trace the letter "Z" with index and middle fingers.

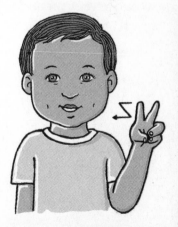

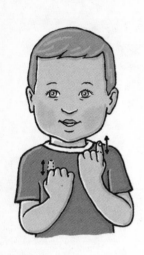

POPCORN

Pop up index fingers like
popcorn popping.

Action Signs

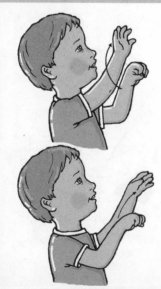

CLIMB

Move curved hands upward
like climbing a ladder.

COOK

Lay hand on the palm of the other hand and then flip it like a pancake.

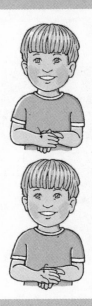

DANCE

Make fingers dance on the palm of the hand.

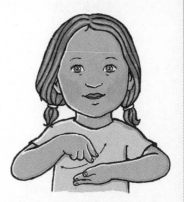

DRAW

Draw on hand with pinkie.

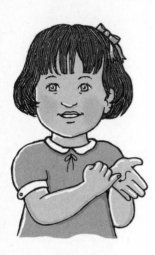

LEARN

Grab information and put
it into your head.

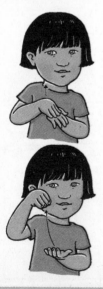

READ

Move index and middle fingers over other hand like reading a book.

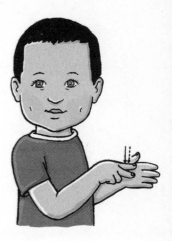

RUN

Pull index finger of one hand with thumb of other hand as both hands move forward.

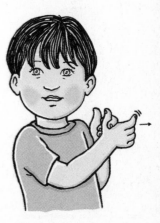

SIT

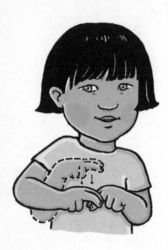

Fold fingers over like legs
sitting on a chair.

SWIM

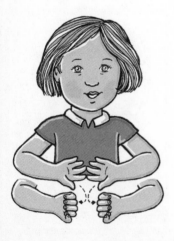

Move hands like you are swimming.

WORK

Tap the back of fist with the other fist.

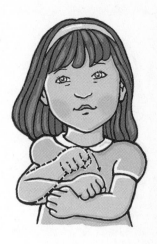

Manners Signs

HELLO

Salute.

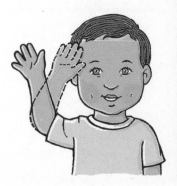

NO

Tap two fingers on thumb.

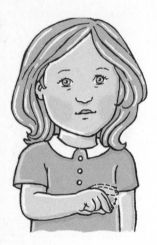

PLEASE

Rub hand over chest in circular motion.

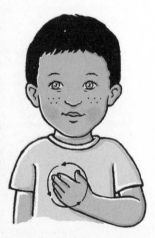

QUIET

Put finger to lips to say "quiet," then move hands out to show that everything gets quiet.

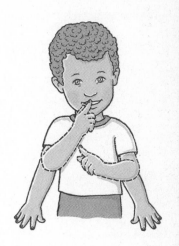

Tip: You can sign just the finger at the lips too, but some moms have found that including the hands moving out helps their children to calm down.

RIGHT

Put index finger to cheek then move down on top of other index finger.

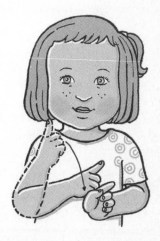

SORRY

Rub fist over heart like
you're really sorry.

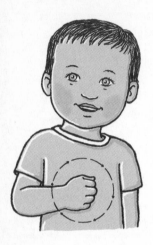

STAY

Stick thumb and pinkie out as
hand moves down firmly.

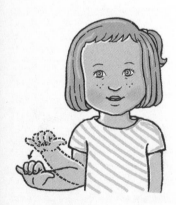

THANK YOU

Touch lips, then move hand out like blowing a kiss.

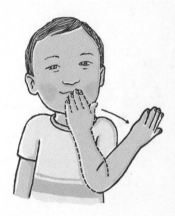

WAIT

Wiggle fingers like you are waiting around.

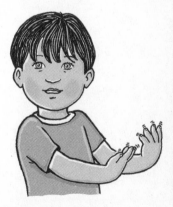

WANT

Grab it and pull it to you.

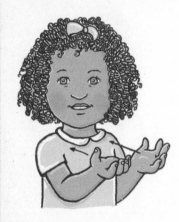

YES

Rock fist like nodding yes.

YOU'RE WELCOME

Move hand from chin to chest.

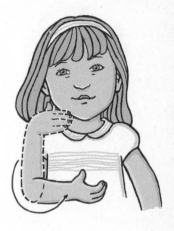

Health and Safety Signs

EARACHE

Touch index fingers together
repeatedly at ear.

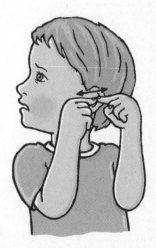

HIT

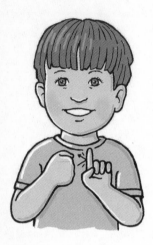

Punch index finger.

MEDICINE

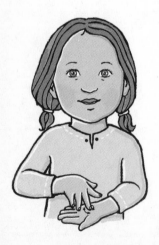

Rock middle finger in center of palm like mixing machine.

Emotions Signs

ANGRY

Move clawlike hand from
angry face to chest.

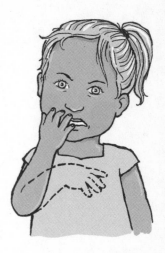

BAD

Move hand from face to
slap the other hand.

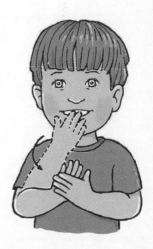

DON'T LIKE

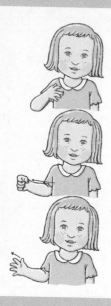

Pull string off shirt and throw away.

FUN

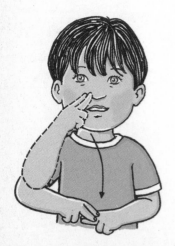

Touch index and middle fingers to nose, then bring them down on to index and middle fingers of the other hand.

GOOD

Move hand from the face to touch the other hand.

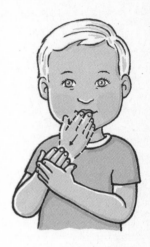

HAPPY

Brush hand up chest repeatedly to show the happiness bubbling over.

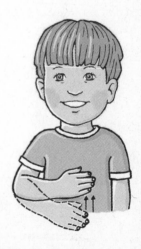

HUNGRY

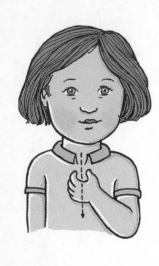

Move curved hand down chest to show food moving down to stomach.

LAUGH

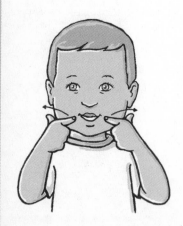

Move index fingers up face repeatedly to show the smile.

LIKE

Pull a string off your shirt.

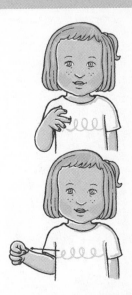

SAD

Move hand over your sad face
in a downward direction.

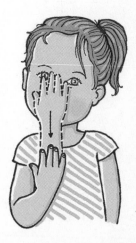

SCARED

Open hand quickly in front
of chest like scared.

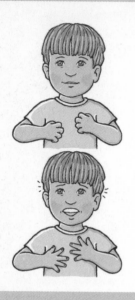

SICK

Touch middle finger to forehead
and stomach and twist.

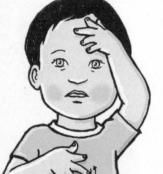

SILLY

Extend thumb and pinkie, then rub thumb across nose a few times.

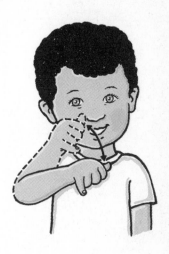

THIRSTY

Run index finger down throat.

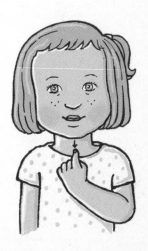

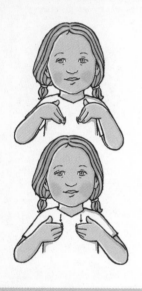

TIRED

Rest fingertips at shoulders, then let them fall forward to show you are tired.

Household Signs

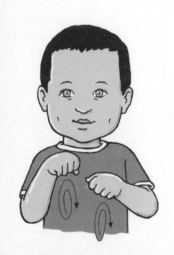

BIKE

Pedal a bike.

FARM

Brush thumb across chin
with fingers open.

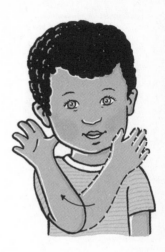

HOUSE

Make a house shape with your hands.

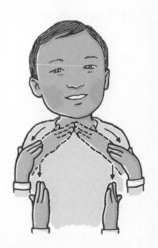

TIME

Tap your watch.

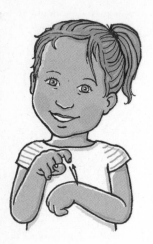

Descriptor Signs

A LOT

Open and close hands repeatedly to show that there is a lot.

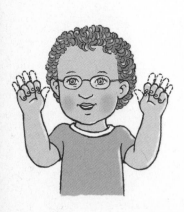

DOWN

Point down.

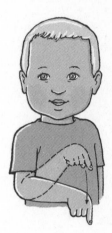

HURRY

Index and middle fingers move
up and down quickly.

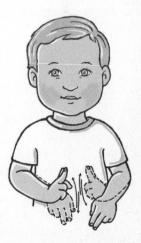

IN/INSIDE

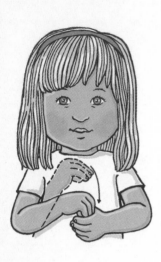

Put something in a container.

LOUD

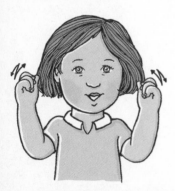

Shake fists at side of head.

SLOW

Move hand slowly up the other hand.

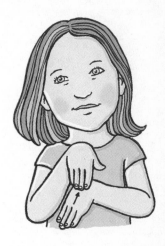

SOUR

Make a sour face and twist
index finger on chin.

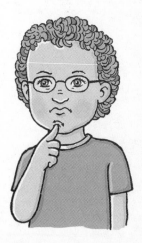

UNDER

Slide hand under the other hand.

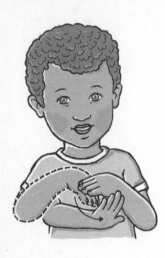

WHAT

Turn both palms up and
gently shake hands.

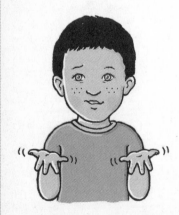

WHERE

Shake finger in the air.

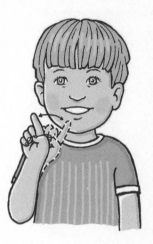

ESSENTIAL SIGNS (NINETEEN TO TWENTY-FOUR MONTHS)

Here are the fifteen essential signs to learn and teach your baby at nineteen to twenty-four months:

1. WAIT (see page 155)
2. PLEASE (see page 152)
3. THANK YOU (see page 155)
4. SORRY (see page 154)
5. QUIET (see page 153)
6. HUNGRY (see page 162)
7. THIRSTY (see page 165)
8. SAD (see page 163)
9. TIRED (see page 166)
10. HAPPY (see page 161)
11. SICK (see page 164)
12. ANGRY (see page 159)
13. BIKE (see page 166)
14. ICE CREAM (see page 143)
15. PIZZA (see page 145)

CHAPTER SIX

NOW WHAT?—TWO YEARS AND BEYOND

NOW THAT YOU ARE EMBARKING on the third year of your child's life, you might be wondering whether signing will continue to play an important role in his development or whether it's not worth the effort anymore. Well, it is worth it, trust me! Most parents and children stop signing somewhere before children are three, but you might be surprised by how long signing can be of use to you. Research shows that children can benefit from signing even in their preschool and kindergarten years. Some schools use signing in their curriculums to help reading and classroom management.

In this chapter, we'll cover the following:

* How your child is developing at two years
* What the long-term effects of signing are
* Why continue to sign
* What to do when your child starts to lose signs
* How to encourage speech

If you are just starting to sign with your child, chances are you are starting now because your child is not speaking yet and you and your pediatrician fear a speech delay. Start signing and watch his language skills develop as he works through his speech issues on his own or with a speech language pathologist (if recommended by your pediatrician). Sometimes it just takes more time to get the right muscle movements to make speech. Read previous chapters to know how to start, but jump in with signs your child is interested in.

SO WHAT'S HAPPENING NOW?

Your child is quite independent now, and she is capable of letting you know what she needs. She is still developing her fine motor skills and will greatly improve her language skills over the next year. She is also working out the rules of social interaction. Signing will help her develop in all of these areas while giving her a way to communicate when she is frustrated or can't yet say the words.

Motor Development

As your child grows, his brain continues to develop, and his fine motor skills improve. Practicing skills reinforces the growth of brain cells and the developing connections between them. Your child will become better at tasks such as dressing, feeding himself, getting a drink, washing his hands, cutting with scissors, drawing with crayons, throwing and kicking a ball, hopping on one foot, pedaling a tricycle, and climbing up and down a small slide. He will also be very proficient at signing by now.

Language Development

By the time she is three, your child will have a vocabulary of at least nine hundred words and use three- to five-word sentences. However, because you signed with your child, her vocabulary might be twice as large as the average child's vocabulary. She will be able to express herself very well.

Cognitive Development

Clearly, you want to do the best you can to create a positive, supportive learning environment for your child—one that optimizes brain growth and all areas of development. Research shows that just playing is the best thing for your child. He is now learning to incorporate his real-life experiences into pretend play. This is his way of figuring out the world around him. The best things you can do are:

* Help him create imaginative games and think of new ways to use toys. Blocks can be food or animals in a pretend zoo.
* Give him time to play by himself. Playing alone gives him a chance to process and understand what he has been doing and learning all day.
* When you read together, ask questions about the book to include him in the story and to make sure he understands.
* Point to the words when you are reading to help him understand the process of reading. Encourage him to sign and say the words he knows.
* Provide materials to scribble, draw, or pretend to write.
* Expose him to books and music, and let him watch you use them in your life. The example you set is very important.

Your child will ask the question "Why?" more frequently. He is naturally curious and wants to learn. Instead of being frustrated when he asks why for the tenth time, see it as an opportunity to engage his brain. Sometimes you can even reverse the question session and ask him why.

How to Manage the "Terrible Twos" with Signs

Two-year-olds are highly involved in their emerging sense of self and cannot fully understand another child's perspective. Additionally, your child is still developing control over her emotions. She may show outbursts of anger and frustration at the same time she is learning to deal with emotions such as shame, wariness, anxiety, fear, pleasure, pride, and joy. Children who have ways to express their emotions with language have an easier time navigating the sometimes explosive emotions of toddler hood. You can help your child by identifying her emotions and giving her words and signs to express them. If she is happy, say "I can see that you are **HAPPY**. You have such a big smile on your face."

Or, if she has hit another child, say and sign "I can see you are **ANGRY**. It is okay to be **ANGRY**, but we don't **HIT**. Use your words instead." Always acknowledge your child's feelings and then offer her concrete consequences for negative behaviors and stick to them. You can also use coping mechanisms such as taking deep breaths, sitting in a comfy chair, or getting a glass of water. Now is a critical time to teach your child how to deal with emotions in addition to validating them. As you give her words to express her emotions, she will gain greater self-control.

> ## THE LONG-TERM EFFECTS OF SIGNING
>
> The positive effects of signing with babies outlast the signs themselves. Signing may even lead to a higher IQ because babies who sign communicate earlier, are exposed to more language opportunities, have an increased vocabulary, and can express complex thoughts earlier. These babies often have better pronunciation and more confidence because they have been initiating conversations from an early age.

WHY CONTINUE TO SIGN?

Because your child can now communicate with both speech and sign, signing takes on a different dimension. Show your child signs for things he is interested in or needs help with. Show him signs for multisyllabic words that are hard to pronounce. By helping him sign the things he wants to talk about and providing him with the ability to express more difficult words, you are empowering him to communicate with you. He will never stop using his hands in some way when he speaks. Even adults use their hands to indicate things such as size, to emphasize words, or to communicate complete thoughts. For example, you might see your friend at a distance and want to tell him to call you, so you sign **TELEPHONE** so that he knows to call you.

If you have another baby, this also gives your child a reason to keep signing: it's something he can show his baby sibling. Put him "in charge" of signing with his brother. Being in charge offers a way to bond with his brother or sister and gives him a sense of his independence and importance in the family. Signing with the second child also helps you as the parent decrease sibling tensions and increase communication bonds. Just as you started with only a few signs with your first child, do the same with his siblings.

HOW TO USE SIGNS TO INTRODUCE THE ALPHABET

Many parents who sign with their children take advantage of this skill to introduce their children to the alphabet. It's a good idea to show your child the manual alphabet (the signs for all the letters) while you are introducing the sounds for the letters and the symbols (written on the page). Just like signing, the alphabet is a system of symbols, so children easily make the leap from hand movements to the alphabet sounds to the alphabet symbols. Singing the alphabet song is a good way to practice too.

If you have not finger-spelled words with your child, now is a good time to do so as well. Start with simple three-letter words and work from there. As Lauri found out, there are other advantages to teaching your child the alphabet through her hands. "I've seen Megan, who is three, get stuck on the LMNO part of the alphabet (speaking), look to my hands for the signs, and then use that to help her remember the English. In English, the LMNO seems like one complicated word. The signs separate them into four letters more visually and seem to help her remember."

As your child progresses and learns more finger spelling, don't be surprised if he asks you to "spell it in your hand." When Alex was three, he came to his mother Nina and asked her how to spell the word **DAD**. "I told him quickly, thinking that he was too young to understand. He then looked at me and said, 'Mom, spell it in your hand.' We had been doing a little bit of finger spelling, but nothing significant. I guess he got the concept and wanted to know how to spell that word. I spelled it for him, and he practiced it for a few minutes. Often, he would ask me to 'spell it in your hand' when he wanted to know how a word was spelled."

Sometimes, your child will even learn to spell words without you knowing it. Barbara says that shortly before her daughter Shira turned two, they were "driving through a small beach town, when we came to a four-way stop. From the backseat, Shira said and finger-spelled, 'S T O P. That spells **STOP**!' I had no idea she could read the sign, much less spell it!"

WHEN YOUR CHILD STOPS SIGNING

You and your child have learned a lot of signs at this point, and the process has hopefully brought you closer together and given you a chance to bond with him. So you might be surprised by how sad you are when your child begins the process of using only speech without signs. Signing has given both of you comfort and peace. But like all things with your child, he is growing in stages and is changing every day. Children stop signing when they feel confident in their ability to get their point across. If your child has advanced so much in his speech that he feels comfortable with speaking only, be happy! You have reached your goal—to bridge the communication gap until your child could speak.

Generally, children stop signing in stages. First, he will sign and say words that he knows how to say. Gradually, the signs will drop off and the words will take over. He will keep a few signs for emphasis or clarification of words he still cannot pronounce. Then, finally, words will take over completely, and he will stop signing unless there is a reason to sign, like a new child or a deaf family member.

Even when your child has a well-developed vocabulary, he might hold on to a few signs that help him communicate better. For example, he might continue to sign **POTTY** so that he can secretly let you know that he has to go potty. Parents report that this is one sign they kept for years after their babies stopped signing as a simple way to ask their child without embarrassing him. Another sign that hangs around for a long time is **HELP**. For the independent souls who don't want anyone to know they need help, this lets you ask them whether they need assistance without saying anything. You also might need to tell your child to **STOP** what he is doing without embarrassing him.

Many children enjoy signing **PLEASE** and **THANK YOU** as a way to show that they really mean what they are saying. Some mothers have found that **WAIT** serves them well when they are in a place such as church or synagogue where their kids need to be quiet and sit still.

Signing also comes in handy when you need to communicate with your mouth full or when you want to communicate when you are on the phone.

HOW TO ENCOURAGE SPEECH

Your goal has always been to help your child learn to use language and to speak. Now that she is well on her way to yapping your ear off, there are ten things you can do to ensure the success of her transition to speech.

1. Do not speak "baby talk" to your child. She is capable of learning *cut*, *scrape*, and *bruise* instead of using *boo-boo* for every injury. When you avoid baby talk, you are extending her vocabulary and increasing her ability to express her needs, wants, and desires.

2. Always respond to your child's attempts to communicate. Don't ignore your child, even if you are involved in something else. Acknowledge him and ask him to **WAIT** for his turn. This is a difficult concept for him to learn, because he is now brimming with desire to communicate.

3. Look directly at your child when you speak (unless driving), speak slowly and clearly, and use complete sentences.

4. Make sure that your requests to your child are simple and direct. Ask one question, wait for her to reply, and then ask her another question. This lets her process each request and respond.

5. Read with your child. Reading exposes him to language he might not hear in daily conversation. Make sure both Mom and Dad have a chance to read to him. If he has an older sibling who can read, enlist his help. Boys especially need to see men reading to them.

6. Expose your child to music, singing, and nursery rhymes. The rhythmic nature of music and rhymes helps your child learn to differentiate sounds and increases her cognitive function.

7. Explain the names and functions of the things your child encounters.

8. Ask your child questions that he can answer. When reading, ask him to find a bird or ask him what color the turtle is. As he gets more sophisticated in his language skills, ask him what is going to happen next in the story.

9. Never make fun of your child's incorrect pronunciation or made-up words. This sends the message that she is doing something wrong and may cause some children to stop progressing verbally. Your child is bound to say funny things such as happycopter (helicopter), boney (bologna), motorbikle (motorcycle), ambliance (ambulance), and blatterfly (butterfly)—these are just a few of the fun things we heard at our house. Enjoy her made-up words and write them down.

10. As he gets older, make up your own stories together. Start a story and

then ask him to add to it. Begin with the plot and ask him to fill in the names and characteristics of the characters in the story. Then add to the story. Once you have added your part, ask him to add more information. You might find that he takes the story in an entirely different direction.

What you are doing now is building your child's lifelong enthusiasm for learning. If he enjoys it now, he will continue to have this experience when he enters school and will become a lifelong learner. You are teaching him knowledge, skills, dispositions, and feelings, and signing helps you do it. You are the most important teacher he will ever have.

FINAL NOTE

This time in your child's life and in your life as a parent is short (even when it feels like it may never end), and your child will never be so innocent or impressionable again. Encourage your baby in everything! Hug her and love her and watch her grow! I know, because my babies have grown, and one is now taller than me. It happens in the blink of an eye. Those grandmothers telling you to enjoy every day are right. Enjoy the journey together, because not only is your child growing, but you are too.

ALL YOU NEED (TWO YEARS AND BEYOND)

- ○ Teach your child signs for words that are hard for him to say.
- ○ Teach your child the alphabet using the manual alphabet.
- ○ Enjoy the signs like PLEASE that your child holds on to.
- ○ Encourage speech through clear and direct communication.
- ○ Engage your child with books and questions so he is able to practice speaking.

QUICK REVIEW OF DEVELOPMENTAL STAGES BY AGE

AGE	MOTOR	LANGUAGE
4–7 months	• reaches for objects • uses finger and thumb to pick up an object • develops a rhythm for feeding, eliminating, sleeping, and being awake • rolls from back to stomach and stomach to back • transfers objects from one hand to the other	• distinguishes sounds • cries in different ways to say she is hurt, wet, hungry, or lonely • makes noises to voice displeasure or satisfaction • babbles expressively as if talking • imitates sounds, actions, and facial expressions made by others • squeals, laughs, babbles, smiles in response • may make first sign
8–12 months	• masters the pincer grasp • continues to explore everything by mouth • crawls well • pulls self to a standing position • stands alone and walks holding onto furniture for support	• makes first sign • says first word • says da-da and ma-ma or equivalent

COGNITIVE	SOCIAL	SIGNING
• recognizes and looks for familiar voices and sounds • learns by using senses like smell, taste, touch, sight, hearing • looks for ball rolled out of sight • searches for toys hidden under a blanket, basket, or container • explores objects by touching, shaking, banging, and mouthing • enjoys dropping objects over edge of chair or crib	• responds to own name • spends a great deal of time watching and observing • responds differently to strangers and family members • likes to be tickled and touched • smiles at own reflection in mirror • raises arms as a sign to be held • recognizes family member names • responds to distress of others by showing distress or crying • shows mild to severe anxiety at separation from parent	• responds to signs with verbal and physical cues • may make one or two signs like **MORE**, **MILK**, or **EAT** • understands as many as fifteen distinct signs
• "dances" or bounces to music • interested in picture books • pays attention to conversations • claps hands and waves bye if prompted • likes to place objects inside one another	• responds to name • likes to watch self in mirror • expresses separation anxiety • pushes away something she does not want	• makes first sign back • masters several signs • may sign two-sign combinations • wants to know the signs for everything he sees

AGE	MOTOR	LANGUAGE
13–18 months	• stands and walks alone • jumps and dances • increases manual dexterity	• responds to simple commands • understands at least 10 to 15 regularly used words; more if she is signing • speaks one or more words • identifies objects correctly
19–24 months	• uses hands more to develop fine motor skills • likes to draw • likes to use a spoon or fork	• speaks several words • may have experienced a language explosion and speak more than 50 words • responds to more complex commands • understands about 200 words
25+ months	• dresses and feeds herself • strings beads, uses paint brushes, cuts with scissors, draws with crayons • throws and kicks a ball, hops on one foot, pedals a tricycle, and climbs up and down a small slide	• understands 400 words at thirty months and up to 800 words at thirty-six months • speaks in three- to five-word sentences • uses past tense correctly most of the time

COGNITIVE	SOCIAL	SIGNING
• recalls things that occurred a few hours or days ago • enjoys repetition as a tool for learning	• imitates adult actions such as drinking from a cup, talking on phone • has a wider range of emotions • has a hard time controlling her emotions	• signs several signs • uses signs to explain what she sees as well as what she needs • may sign and speak to communicate a thought
• learns through experience more than stories • understands that symbols stand for objects • understands symbolic thought and pretend play	• imitates adult actions such as drinking from a cup, talking on phone • can play alone for longer periods of time • may become possessive of toys • may be able to learn the beginning of sharing	• signs and speaks at the same time • gradually drops signs for the words she can speak clearly
• asks why frequently • asks questions when you read books • may recognize letters and some simple words	• plays by herself • plays imaginative games and thinks of new ways to use toys • can share toys • learning to control very strong emotions • pushes boundaries to understand the rules	• signs and speaks at the same time • gradually drops signs for the words she can speak clearly • may keep a few signs she especially loves

SIGNING WITH CHILDREN WHO HAVE SPECIAL NEEDS

PARENTS WHOSE CHILDREN ARE NOT speaking on schedule often worry whether their child is delayed, because, as noted at the beginning of the book, language is the primary tool that we use to understand others (*receptive language*) and to be understood by others (*expressive language*). We communicate with others using words, signs, or writing, and *language* includes the types of words we use, how many words we use, how we put the words together to form thoughts, and so on. *Speech*, on the other hand, is how we pronounce words. Children can have a delay in either speech or language or both.

Children with *mixed language delay*—a delay in understanding how language works—often have difficulty with both receptive and expressive language. For these children, using signs in addition to speech can be particularly useful for enhancing receptive language skills (understanding others). The visual cues that signs provide help children better understand spoken language, while also providing them with vocabulary they can use.

Children with *expressive language delay* have receptive language skills appropriate for their age but are not using the average number of words and are considered late talkers. Late talkers can become easily frustrated, because they know and understand the same level of language as their peers but just aren't talking yet. Signing gives these children a functional means to communicate while working toward spoken language. More than 80 percent of children who are late talkers at twenty-four months old catch up by age three with no intervention. But it can be challenging for you and your child to wait that long. Using signs can alleviate most of that frustration, because you have a communication tool that your child can use to express wants and needs.

Speech delay is most often caused by physical issues such as a lisp or stuttering, or by articulation or phonological difficulties (difficulty learning associations between the visual forms of letters or pairs of letters and the sounds that they represent). Sometimes extra fluid in the ear can impair hearing and also cause speech delay, and the delay will resolve itself once your child can hear how speech is made. For more information on speech and language delay, see the American Speech-Language-Hearing Association (ASHA) website (www.asha.org). Always consult with your pediatrician as well.

SPECIAL NEEDS AND SIGNING

There are several special needs conditions that cause children to have either a language delay or a speech delay or both. The following is a list of conditions and how children with them may benefit from using sign language:

- **Apraxia/dyspraxia:** When signing is used with toddlers and preschoolers who have apraxia, it takes the pressure off verbal language and relieves the frustration associated with speaking, since apraxia affects coordination of the muscles. It also makes children more willing to try to talk, which can reduce aggression associated with this frustration. For more information, see www.apraxia-kids.org.

- **Down syndrome:** Children with Down syndrome often do not begin using verbal language until after their second birthday. This makes them perfect candidates for the use of signing. Many children with Down syndrome develop functional communication skills and do not need to rely on signing after five or six years old. Others, due to cognitive and motor delays, will rely on the use of signing throughout life to augment their verbal communication skills.

- **Autism and pervasive developmental disorders:** Children with autism often have difficulty not just using words, but also with the social aspect of language. Signing can help these children communicate functionally with others. For a child with autism to use signing, she must be intentional in her communication—she must be trying to send you a message. She must also have joint attention—the ability to shift her eye gaze between you and the object you are talking about. You can pair signing with other communication techniques used with children with autism such as the Picture Exchange Communication System (PECS). Then you have a way to communicate when you don't have the cards you created for PECS around, because you always have your hands with you.

- **Cognitive delay:** Children with cognitive delays tend to develop more slowly in many areas of development, especially thinking, play, and speech and language skills. They will follow the same sequence of development as other children, but at a slower rate. They often have shorter attention spans and are easily distracted. Behavior can become a problem, because they know what they want or need but do not have the skills to tell you yet. Signing can be used to help them with both receptive and expressive language.

- **Medically fragile:** Children who are born premature or with extensive medical problems often show delays in their development during the first two years of life. Long hospital stays, surgical procedures, and medical equipment may interfere with a family's ability to interact with and nurture their child. Signing can help alleviate the stress of not being able to communicate during the time of delay.

- **Cleft palate:** Children with a cleft palate are often very difficult to understand until palatal repair is complete. While the initial repair of the palate is usually done prior to the first birthday, additional surgeries may be needed to obtain intelligible speech. Signing offers children an opportunity to express themselves without the frustration of not being understood.

- **Tracheotomy:** Children and adults with tracheotomies cannot make their voice work without a special valve in the trach tube. Many children do not have access to the valve because of ongoing respiratory issues. By using signing, you can minimize delays in language by giving your child a means to communicate and develop language skills. She will then learn to talk when the trach is removed or the special valve is added to the trach tube.

There are many other genetic and medical conditions that affect a child's motor skills and communication and cognitive abilities. When signing with children who have special needs, be aware of the symptoms and developmental concerns associated with the particular diagnosis. Some conditions affect cognitive and language skills while others may impact vision or hearing. Talk with your medical professionals about using signing.

MODIFYING SIGNING FOR CHILDREN WITH SPECIAL NEEDS

When you are signing with a child who has special needs, you will need to adapt your strategies and your approach to meet her abilities and needs. Read *Baby Signing Essentials* and then keep several things in mind as you modify your signing experience.

Don't Be Afraid to Sign!

Children with special needs often require things be tweaked a bit to suit them. As you read through this book, think about how the suggestions might apply to your child. What would you need to change? Nothing about signing with babies is set in stone, so feel free to adapt it to your needs and the needs of your child. You know his strengths and abilities best.

If your child is severely delayed, before he can sign, he must be able to bring his hands together at midline so that he can form signs, and he must understand object permanence to know something exists when it is out of sight. If your child has not reached these milestones yet, he may do so later and be able to sign in the future. Today, caregivers in adult Down syndrome programs are introducing signs to their adult patients with some success, so signing does not have to occur at a specific age to have benefit for people with special needs.

Always Speak When Signing

You should always speak when you sign. Of course, this is also true when you sign with hearing children who are developing normally, but sometimes people forget to speak with children who have special needs. Because it might take children with special needs longer to communicate back, parents and caregivers might fall into a pattern of silence. However, the more exposure to spoken language you give to children with special needs, the better chance they have of developing the ability to speak.

Watch for Approximations

All children approximate signs while gaining fine motor skills. However, children with special needs may always approximate their signs because their motor skills are affected by their condition. For example, children with Down syndrome may grossly approximate signs due to delays in fine motor skills or may sign in the wrong location due to gross motor difficulties. Kim Fries, a speech-language pathologist and signing instructor, worked with an eighteen-month-old boy with Down syndrome who sat independently but quite wobbly. His signs had accurate hand shapes and movements but were signed next to his leg. Because he spent so much energy trying to stay upright, he could not move his hand to his chest or face to sign without falling over.

Sign Specific and Concrete Signs

Instead of using such general signs as **MORE**, **EAT**, and **DRINK**, teach specific signs such as **MILK**, **CRACKER**, or **BANANA**. This will help you avoid a situation where your child is asking for **MORE** and you are guessing what it is that she wants. With normally developing children, this is not usually a problem, but with children who have language difficulties, it can be. The more specific the signs are that your child learns, the less chance of confusion and frustration. Additionally, it is better to teach signs for concrete things rather than abstract concepts, because children with special needs might not be able to make the abstract connections.

Concentrate on Signs That Are Functional and Motivating

Concentrate on functional signs that your child will be able to use immediately to get things he wants or needs. Using signs for things that your child needs will motivate him to learn to sign. Foods, favorite toys or activities, and people are great signs to begin with. As discussed before, avoid general signs such as **MORE**, **EAT**, **DRINK**, or **PLAY** until your child has established a core vocabulary to avoid having to figure out what your child specifically wants.

Don't Expect Results Overnight

Your child might take a long time to sign back, so all guesses on a timeline for communication are off. There is no way to estimate how long it might take. However, it is worth the wait and the effort to have your child be able to communicate. Before she can sign, she will probably respond to you in other ways, so look for other signs of recognition such as grunts, eye movements, changes in demeanor, or even changes in posture.

Michelle teaches children with severe disabilities in ages ranging from three to five years. One child with severe autism shakes and has tics but has learned to sign a few signs at home and at school (she has taught the entire class **HELP**, **SHARE**, **SORRY**, **PLEASE**, **MORE**, **EAT**, **DRINK**, **WATER**, and the signs for colors). She says that after working with this boy for a very long time, she could see "the light go on in his eyes. He learned the sign **FRIEND**, and he really got it. When I can get his attention and sign to him, he is able to focus on me—his tics subside—and he is able to communicate. It is hard to get through to him, but it is worth it when you see the light go on—it is a heavenly thing!"

Look for Help If You Need It

If you have not already done so, seek help from your local resources. Work with a speech-language pathologist (SLP) or an occupational therapist (OT) who understands how much signing can help children with special needs. It is a growing trend that both SLPs and OTs use signing in their therapy. Ask at the schools your child will attend whether they encourage signing. More and more schools are helping children by using signing in the classroom. If your school does not use signing now, ask them whether they would be open to having your child use signing with the teacher. You could spend some extra time with the teacher, helping her to see the benefits of signing.

Keep It Fun!

Make sure you don't get stressed out and don't push your child. Keep it fun, and you will both have a better experience. As with most things you want to teach your special needs child, keeping the stress down and the situation fun will yield better results than pressuring your child to sign back. Use games and songs and other motivations to teach her the signs.

A FINAL NOTE ON SIGNING WITH CHILDREN WHO HAVE SPECIAL NEEDS

You have been blessed with a special child. Even though it takes more effort to sign with your child, the results will be worth it. As Jason found out, signing may sometimes be the only effective way of communicating and helping your child: "After my son Austin was diagnosed with autism at three, we got him into a special school where teachers used signing to reinforce verbal cues. Austin is now five and in a special kindergarten class where they don't seem to use the signing as much, and we have kind of slacked off. About six months ago, he was having a meltdown. After repeatedly telling him that we were all done and to stop, something in the back of my mind told me to get his attention through signs instead. So I said and signed **STOP**, **LOOK**, **LISTEN**, **SIT**, and **ALL DONE**. The meltdown ended immediately. He wiped his face and gave me a hug and very calmly, with two signs, told me **MORE JUICE**. It clicked with him that we can communicate.

"Ever since that day, I have worked with him and continue to learn new signs as needed to communicate with him. If a meltdown starts, 95 percent of the time, it can be solved in some manner through signing and verbal communication together. The other 5 percent of the time, I understand the need and just don't give in. Signing has been nothing but a blessing for my autistic son—a blessing that opened a door into his world and allows for him to tell me what he can't put into words."

ALPHABETICAL LIST
OF ALL SIGNS

INDEX

V

Z

ABOUT THE AUTHOR

NANCY CADJAN IS THE CREATOR of Sign Babies ASL Flash Cards, which have sold over eighty thousand sets, and the author of the award-winning book *Baby Signing 1-2-3*. Nancy hosts two podcasts called Babies and Moms: Birth and Beyond and The MOM Podcast. She also blogs on parenting topics. She lives with her husband and two children in Utah, where they enjoy skiing and biking.